Rabies in Man and Animals

Sudhi Ranjan Garg

Rabies in Man and Animals

Springer

Sudhi Ranjan Garg
Veterinary Public Health &
Epidemiology
Lala Lajpat Rai University of Veterinary
and Animal Sciences
Hisar, Haryana, India

ISBN 978-81-322-1604-9 ISBN 978-81-322-1605-6 (eBook)
DOI 10.1007/978-81-322-1605-6
Springer New Delhi Heidelberg New York Dordrecht London

Printed on acid-free paper

Springer is part of Springer Science+Business Media (www.springer.com)

To my beloved wife, Meenakshi

Preface

Rabies is among the oldest zoonotic diseases that are transmissible from animals to human beings. All mammals are believed to be susceptible to rabies and the transmission of infection usually occurs through the bite of an infected host. With only Antarctica as the rabies-free continent, the disease has a near cosmopolitan distribution, although several isolated rabies-free countries do exist. The infection in unvaccinated humans is almost invariably fatal, although a few cases of people surviving confirmed rabies infection have been reported. Despite being a vaccine-preventable disease, rabies causes deaths of more people than many other common infectious diseases worldwide. Rabies is uniformly fatal in domestic and wild animals.

The highest incidence of human rabies fatalities is encountered in the developing countries, mainly in Asia and Africa including India. Domestic dogs remain the major reservoirs in such countries while many developed nations have successfully controlled canine rabies through systematic rabies prevention and control programmes. Rabies can be successfully prevented with the modern highly potent cell culture vaccines, but the disease still continues to haunt mankind globally. Even in the developed countries which have been able to eliminate human rabies, the virus continues to circulate in dogs and wildlife reservoirs necessitating constant surveillance and monitoring.

The resource constraint is mainly responsible for the grim situation in the developing countries but the picture is not very bright even at places where well-equipped laboratories and trained staff exist, usually due to the low priority accorded to rabies control programmes. The misconceptions and lack of awareness among health professionals, veterinarians, civic bodies and the public further aggravate the problem. It has been noted that most humans die due to rabies because they fail to get timely and appropriate post-exposure treatment, particularly in rural and remote areas. Many dog bites, especially in children, are either ignored or reported late which leads to completely missing the life-saving post-exposure treatment or delay in its administration. Incomplete or faulty treatment due to ignorance and other factors also compounds the problem.

In rabies-endemic countries, the disease can be effectively targeted by using the models and guidelines of previous successful rabies control programmes. This book provides an insight into the risk analysis and epidemiology of rabies in different parts of the world and elaborates the challenges in rabies control along with cost-effective ways to overcome the constraints. Apart from updating the knowledge and skills of the health professionals and veterinarians, the book will be quite useful in educating people. The illustrations and simple language in the book are expected to assist in evolving practical strategies for control and eventual elimination of rabies in human beings and animals through intersectoral coordination.

Hisar, India Sudhi Ranjan Garg

Acknowledgements

I wish to express my deep sense of regard and indebtedness to the following organizations and individuals for their able guidance and untiring support in providing an excellent academic environment in working on the book:

Association for Prevention and Control of Rabies in India
Blueprint for Rabies Prevention and Control
Centers for Disease Control and Prevention, USA (CDC)
Dr. F. A. Murphy, University of Texas Medical Branch, Galveston, Texas
Dr. Richard Hunt, University of South Carolina School of Medicine
Global Alliance for Rabies Control
Health Protection Agency, UK
Health Protection Scotland
National Association of State Public Health Veterinarians, USA
National Centre for Disease Control, New Delhi
Public Health Image Library, CDC
Rabies Bulletin Europe
The Center for Food Security and Public Health, Iowa State University
U.S. Department of Agriculture, Animal and Plant Health Inspection Service
WHO Collaboration Centre for Rabies Surveillance and Research, Germany
World Health Organization
World Organisation for Animal Health (OIE)

Contents

Abbreviations

ABC	Animal birth control
ABC Rules	Animal Birth Control (Dogs) Rules, 2001
ABC-AR	Animal birth control and anti-rabies
ABLV	Australian bat lyssavirus
ACIP	United States Advisory Committee on Immunization Practices
APCRI	Association for Prevention and Control of Rabies in India
ARAV	Aravan virus
AREB	Asian Rabies Expert Bureau
AWBI	Animal Welfare Board of India
BHK	Baby hamster kidney
CDC	Centers for Disease Control and Prevention
CFIA	Canadian Food Inspection Agency
CNS	Central nervous system
CSF	Cerebrospinal fluid
CVS	Challenge virus standard
DALY	Disability-adjusted life year
dRIT	Direct rapid immunohistochemical test
DUVV	Duvenhage virus
EBLV	European bat lyssaviruses
ELISA	Enzyme-linked immunosorbent assay
ERIG	Equine rabies immunoglobulin
FAO	Food and Agriculture Organization of the United Nations
FAT	Fluorescent antibody test
FAVN	Fluorescent antibody virus neutralization
FITC	Fluorescein isothiocyanate
GARC	Global Alliance for Rabies Control
HDCV	Human diploid cell vaccine
HEP	High egg passage
HRIG	Human rabies immunoglobulin
ICTV	International Committee on Taxonomy of Viruses
IDRV	Intradermal rabies vaccination
IFA	Indirect fluorescent antibody test
IHC	Immunohistochemistry
IRKV	Irkut virus
KHUV	Khujand virus
LBV	Lagos bat virus

LEP	Low egg passage
MAb	Monoclonal antibodies
MI	Mouse inoculation
MNT	Mouse neutralization test
MOKV	Mokola virus
NASPHV	National Association of State Public Health Veterinarians
NGO	Non-governmental organization
NICD	National Institute of Communicable Diseases
NIH	National Institute of Health
OIE	World Organisation for Animal Health
ORV	Oral rabies vaccination
PAHO	Pan American Health Organization
PCECV	Purified chick embryo cell vaccine
PCR-ELISA	Polymerase chain reaction-enzyme linked immunosorbent assay
PDEV	Purified duck embryo vaccine
PEP	Post-exposure prophylaxis
PVRV	Purified Vero cell rabies vaccine
RABV	Rabies virus
RFFIT	Rapid fluorescent focus inhibition test
RIG	Rabies immunoglobulin
RIT	Rapid immunohistochemical test
RNA	Ribonucleic acid
RREID	Rapid rabies enzyme immunodiagnosis
RT	Reverse transcriptase
RT-PCR	Reverse transcription polymerase chain reaction
RVA	Rabies vaccine adsorbed
SHIBV	Shimoni bat virus
SOP	Standard operating procedures
SPCA	Society for Prevention of Cruelty to Animals
TVR	Trap-vaccinate-release
US	United States
VNA	Virus neutralization antibodies
WCBV	West Caucasian bat virus
WHO	World Health Organization

1 Introduction

Abstract

Rabies, also known as hydrophobia in man, is among the most dreadful zoonotic diseases. It affects the central nervous system of humans and warm-blooded animals. The disease is transmitted from animal to animal and from animal to man through saliva. Despite being vaccine preventable, rabies kills more than 55,000 people worldwide every year apart from causing huge loss of domestic animals. Most human rabies deaths occur in Asia and Africa; India alone shares 36 % of the global burden. Rabies virus is present on all continents except Antarctica. Many strains of rabies virus and many animal species are involved in the maintenance and transmission of the disease. All mammalian species including nonhuman primates and humans are affected. Major reservoir hosts vary with the area. Canine rabies predominates in most of the developing countries. More than 90 % of cases of human rabies are transmitted by dogs which is a major concern for public health in these countries. However, the disease is present mainly in wildlife hosts in some other regions. Besides canines, skunks, mongooses, raccoons, and bats, domestic animals including cattle, sheep, goats, horses, and swine are also susceptible.

1.1 Background

Rabies is regarded as one of the most important zoonotic diseases in the world. Commonly known as hydrophobia in man, it is a viral disease that affects the central nervous system (CNS) of humans and warm-blooded animals. Rabies is transmitted from animal to animal and from animal to man through saliva. Animal bites introduce the virus into muscle and nerve ending-rich tissues from which it penetrates into nerve cells where it replicates and progressively travels through the spinal cord to the brain. This process usually requires weeks or even months, depending upon the distance from the site of the bite to the brain. The disease causes hydrophobia in man, hallucinations, aggressive behaviour, and paralysis, eventually leading to coma and death. Once the symptoms appear, rabies is nearly always fatal.

Rabies has been recognised for centuries. The word rabies is derived from the Latin word *rabere*, which means to be mad, to rage, or to rave. The word might be having roots in a Sanskrit word *rabhas* that means to do violence. The first written description of rabies in the literature is cited in the Babylon Codex (23 centuries BC). Dog owners in

S.R. Garg, *Rabies in Man and Animals*, DOI 10.1007/978-81-322-1605-6_1,

the Babylonian city of Eshnunna were fined heavily for deaths caused by their dogs biting the people. Democritus, a Greek philosopher, recorded a case of canine rabies in 500 BC. In 400 BC, Aristotle wrote that 'dogs suffer from the madness. This causes them to become very irritable and all animals they bite become diseased'. Rabies is now present on all continents except in Antarctica, but more than 95 % of human deaths occur in Asia and Africa. The disease primarily infects domestic and wild animals and is transmitted to humans through close contact with infected saliva via bites or scratches, mainly of dogs.

In 1885, Louis Pasteur obtained his first success against rabies through postexposure vaccination (Bourhy et al. 2010), but even more than 125 years later, the disease still continues to affect mankind, especially in developing countries in Africa, Asia, and Latin America. Despite the existence of effective vaccines for both human and veterinary use, it is estimated that rabies kills more than 55,000 people worldwide every year besides causing huge loss of domestic animals. Based on the disability-adjusted life year (DALY) score, it has been estimated that deaths due to rabies would be responsible for 1.74 million DALYs lost each year in Africa and Asia (Knobel et al. 2005). An additional loss of 0.04 million DALYs may occur due to the side effects from nerve tissue vaccines. The estimated annual cost of rabies including costs of postexposure prophylaxis (PEP), expenses on rabies control in dogs, and livestock losses has been put at US$583.5 million.

The true global impact of rabies may be much more. Human mortality data alone may not give the real picture of the quantum of the risk of exposure to rabies from animals. The incidence of rabies might be largely underestimated due to poor reporting and lack of diagnostic facilities and surveillance, particularly in the developing countries. While all mammalian species, including nonhuman primates and humans, are believed to be susceptible to rabies, it is primarily not a disease of humans. Human infection is incidental to the reservoir of disease in wild and domestic animals. In the natural sense, rabies is a disease of wild carnivores involving dogs, cats, wolves, foxes, coyotes, jackals, raccoons, skunks, and bats as reservoirs and vectors. Therefore, a more accurate projection of the impact of rabies on public health should include an estimate of the extent to which the animal population is affected and the number and distribution of cases of rabies in domestic animals (CDC 2012).

1.2 Geographical Distribution

Rabies virus is known to be endemic in at least 150 countries. While in some regions, the disease is present mainly in wildlife hosts, rabies in domestic dogs is of major concern for public health in many developing countries. Some countries including the UK, Ireland, Sweden, Norway, Iceland, Japan, Australia, New Zealand, Singapore, most of Malaysia, Papua New Guinea, the Pacific Islands, and some islands in Indonesia have been free of the classical rabies virus for many years (CFSPH 2009), but the number and size of rabies-free countries, territories, or areas are small in comparison to those of rabies-affected areas. Adequate surveillance, import regulations, and vaccination programmes reduce the occurrence of cases of rabies in man and animals. Some countries have succeeded in controlling and even eradicating the disease by implementing vigilant control measures; however, the rabies-free status of any country, area, and population may change due to reintroduction of virus. For example, rabies was introduced in the year 2008 into the island of Bali (Indonesia), which had been free of rabies for many years. A lack of surveillance allowed the import of an unvaccinated rabid dog to Bali from Flores, a distant island where canine rabies was similarly introduced in 1997 and has since become endemic (Clifton 2010).

According to the World Health Organization (WHO) estimates, the number of human rabies deaths in Asia is more than 31,000 per year, of which more than 20,000 occur in India alone. India thus accounts for 36 % of the global human rabies death burden. Rabies is endemic in India except in Andaman and Nicobar and Lakshadweep islands, which are historically known to be rabies-free. The extent of rabies burden among

Table 1.1 Rabies outbreaks in animals in India reported to OIE (1996 to 2004) (OIE 2011)

Year	Species	Number of Outbreaks	Cases	Deaths
1996	Cattle	16	286	286
	Dogs	35	84	84
1997	Cattle	12	70	70
	Dogs	25	35	35
	Sheep/goats	1	Information not available	
1998	Cattle	10	137	137
	Buffaloes	Information not available		
	Dogs	40	200	200
	Cats	0	0	0
	Sheep/goats	0	0	0
1999	Cattle	21	55	55
	Buffaloes	Information not available		
	Dogs	13	29	29
2000	Cattle	23	62	62
	Dogs	11	32	32
2001	Cattle	89	297	297
	Buffaloes	5	41	41
	Dogs	20	75	75
	Sheep/goats	15	74	74
2002	Cattle	126	420	420
	Buffaloes	2	16	16
	Dogs	14	214	214
	Sheep/goats	5	7	7
2003	Cattle	51	130	130
	Buffaloes	3	15	15
	Dogs	7	20	20
	Equidae	2	3	3
	Sheep/goats	4	9	9
2004	Cattle	29	85	85
	Buffaloes	1	1	1
	Dogs	4	12	12
	Sheep/goats	2	54	54
1996 to 2004	Total	586	2,463	2,463

animals in the country is not exactly known, but the incidence of the disease is quite high and the disease is frequently encountered in different parts of the country. The description of the outbreaks of rabies in animals during the years 1996 to 2004 reported to the World Organisation for Animal Health (OIE) is given in Table 1.1. India reported 586 outbreaks among different species of animals leading to death of 2,463 animals during this period. Subsequently, 398 outbreaks of rabies in animals were reported during the period 2005 to 2011, the geographical distribution of which is given in Table 1.2. Many areas of the country did not report any case during this long period of 7 years despite the endemic status of rabies there. The actual numbers, therefore,

Table 1.2 Number of outbreaks of rabies in animals reported from India to OIE (2005 to 2011) (OIE 2013)

State/union territory	2005	2006	2007	2008	2009	2010	2011	Total
Andhra Pradesh	3	–	7	1	–	–	2	13
Arunachal Pradesh	–	–	–	–	–	2	–	2
Goa	1	1	–	–	–	–	–	2
Gujarat	1	1	1	–	5	–	–	8
Himachal Pradesh	1	–	–	–	–	1	–	2
Jammu and Kashmir	2	5	6	6	6	–	–	25
Karnataka	–	–	6	15	9	9	7	46
Kerala	3	–	–	–	1	–	–	4
Madhya Pradesh	–	–	–	1	–	–	–	1
Maharashtra	–	–	–	–	7	1	–	8
Manipur	–	–	–	1	–	9	7	17
Meghalaya	–	–	–	2	42	22	17	83
Mizoram	–	–	–	–	3	–	–	3
Nagaland	2	–	3	10	8	8	1	32
Orissa (Odisha)	–	–	4	5	9	–	–	18
Pondicherry	2	–	–	–	1	4	1	8
Rajasthan	–	–	–	–	2	–	–	2
Tamil Nadu	–	–	–	–	1	–	–	1
Tripura	–	–	–	2	2	6	28	38
Uttar Pradesh	–	–	–	–	–	4	26	30
West Bengal	16	10	16	4	1	4	3	54
Jharkhand	–	–	–	–	–	1	–	1
Total	31	17	43	47	97	71	92	398

may be substantially higher, considering the possibility of underreporting due to weak rabies surveillance and inadequate reporting mechanism in the country.

1.3 Reservoirs and Host Range

All mammals are susceptible to rabies virus. As there are many strains of rabies virus, many animal species are involved in the maintenance and transmission of the disease. Each rabies virus strain is maintained in nature in particular animal species. The animal hosts include members of the family Canidae (dogs, jackals, coyotes, wolves, foxes, and raccoon dogs), Mustelidae (skunks, martens, weasels, and stoats), Viverridae (mongooses and meerkats), and Procyonidae (raccoons) and the order Chiroptera (bats). The important reservoir hosts vary with the area (CFSPH 2009).

Canine rabies predominates in most of the developing countries of Central and South America, Africa, and Asia, which share the greater burden of human rabies. More than 90 % of cases of human rabies are transmitted by dogs (WHO 2012). Apart from dogs, wildlife hosts are also present in these regions. Jackals, bat-eared foxes, and mongooses are involved in rabies transmission in Africa, particularly in the southeastern part of the continent. In Central and South America, rabies has been reported in wolves, coyotes, skunks, and foxes while mongooses are also important in the Caribbean. Red and arctic foxes, raccoon dogs, mongooses, and jackals are the rabies reservoir hosts in parts of Asia, and red foxes and golden jackals in the Middle East. A variety of bat species have been shown to harbour rabies or rabies-related viruses in Africa, Australia, Central and Southeast Asia, Europe, and most of the Americas (CFSPH 2009; WHO 2012).

The canine rabies variant is well controlled in the United States (USA), Canada, and Europe, and it may no longer be circulating or circulates only at low levels in some areas. In parts of Canada and the USA, skunk, raccoon, and fox rabies is widely prevalent. In North America, maintenance hosts for rabies virus include insectivorous bats, striped skunks, raccoons, coyotes, and various species of foxes. Red foxes, insectivorous bats, wolves, and raccoon dogs appear to be important hosts in Europe (CFSPH 2009; WHO 2012). Infected wildlife species, including bats, can transmit rabies to humans, but the overall number of such cases remains limited compared with the annual number of human deaths caused by dog-transmitted rabies.

Domesticated animals like cattle, sheep, goats, horses, and swine are also susceptible which may contribute in maintaining rabies in nature.

References

Bourhy H, Perrot A, Cavaillon JM (2010) Rabies. In: Arstentein AW (ed) Vaccines: a biography. Springer, New York, pp 73–85

CDC (2012) Rabies. Centers for Disease Control and Prevention. http://www.cdc.gov/rabies/. Accessed 30 Mar 2012

CFSPH (2009) Rabies. The Center for Food Security and Public Health, Iowa State University. Iowa. http://www.cfsph.iastate.edu/Factsheets/pdfs/rabies.pdf. Accessed 15 Mar 2011

Clifton M (2010) How not to fight a rabies epidemic: a history in Bali. Asian Biomed 4:663–670

Knobel DL, Cleaveland S, Coleman PG, Fevre EM, Meltzer MI, Miranda ME, Shaw A, Zinsstag J, Meslin FX (2005) Re-evaluating the burden of rabies in Africa and Asia. Bull WHO 83:360–368

OIE (2011) HANDISTATUS II. World Organisation for Animal Health, Paris, France. http://www.oie.int/animal-health-in-the-world/the-world-animal-health-information-system/data-before-2005-handistatus/. Accessed 15 Mar 2011

OIE (2013) World Animal Health Information Database (WAHID) Interface. World Organisation for Animal Health. http://web.oie.int/wahis/public.php?page=home. Accessed 25 May 2013

WHO (2012) Rabies. World Health Organization. www.who.int. Accessed 10 Mar 2012

2 Causation of Disease

Abstract

Rabies viruses consist of a group of negative-strand RNA neurotropic viruses of the genus *Lyssavirus*. The classical rabies virus found worldwide is responsible for classical rabies that constitutes a vast majority of rabies cases. Other lyssaviruses appear to have more restricted geographical and host range. All species of mammals are susceptible but only a few species are important as major reservoirs. The virus is transmitted between mammals usually through saliva and animal bites. Contact with infectious saliva or neurological tissues, through mucous membrane or abraded skin, may also cause infection. Dogs are the main hosts in Asia and Africa while wild animals act as major hosts in Europe, North America, and Australia, from which the disease spills over to domestic animals and humans. Certain categories of people such as those living in or travelling to the rabies-endemic areas or those occupationally exposed to animals, animal bites, or infected material face greater risk of infection. Inadequate medical facilities and unavailability of vaccines and immunoglobulin in rural high-risk areas make the residents and travellers more prone to the disease.

2.1 Etiological Agent

As early as the first century AD, the infectivity of the saliva of rabid dogs was described by Cardanus, a Roman writer. He described the saliva from a rabid dog as a *virus* – the Latin word for poison. Historically, Celsus, a physician and naturalist, used the term rabies 'virus' (but in the sense of poison or venom) and emphasised that the bites of all animals that contained virus were dangerous to man and to other animals (Smithcors 1958; Mutinelli et al. 2004). Pliny attributed canine rabies to the existence of a small worm ('lyssa'), situated under the fraenum of the dog's tongue (Théodoridès 1986; Blancou 2004).

Rabies is caused by negative-strand ribonucleic acid (RNA) neurotropic viruses of the genus *Lyssavirus* in the family *Rhabdoviridae* and order *Mononegavirales*. The name Rhabdo comes from the Greek word and identifies the characteristic bullet or rod shape of the viruses (Fig. 2.1). Rabies viruses consist of a group of viruses including several recently identified bat lyssaviruses responsible for causing encephalitis. Based on demarcation criteria such as genetic distance and antigenic patterns in reactions with

S.R. Garg, *Rabies in Man and Animals*, DOI 10.1007/978-81-322-1605-6_2,

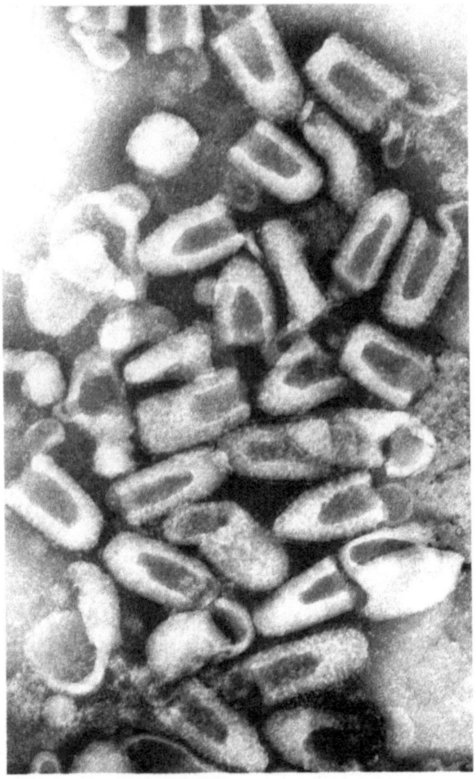

Fig. 2.1 Rabies virus, purified from an infected cell culture. Negatively stained virions showing characteristic '*bullet shape*'. Magnification approximately ×70,000 (Murphy 2012)

panels of antinucleocapsid monoclonal antibodies, the International Committee on Taxonomy of Viruses (ICTV) has delineated the genus *Lyssavirus* into 12 species as of 2011 shown in Table 2.1 (ICTV 2012). This demarcation is further supported by geographical distribution and host range as depicted in the table (Rabies Bulletin Europe 2012).

A newly identified lyssavirus, Bokeloh bat lyssavirus detected in bats (*Myotis nattereri*) distributed in Europe, has not yet been classified (Freuling et al. 2011; Rabies Bulletin Europe 2012). In another recent report, evidence in support of a novel lyssavirus was obtained from brain samples of an African civet (nocturnal, catlike animal) in Tanzania (Marston et al. 2012). Results of phylogenetic analysis of nucleoprotein gene sequences from representative lyssavirus species and this novel lyssavirus provided strong empirical evidence that this is a new lyssavirus species, designated Ikoma lyssavirus.

Lyssavirus species segregate into two or more phylogroups. Phylogroup 1 includes Rabies virus (RABV), Duvenhage virus (DUVV); European bat lyssaviruses, types 1 and 2 (EBLV-1 and EBLV-2, respectively); Australian bat lyssavirus (ABLV); Aravan virus (ARAV); Khujand virus (KHUV); and Irkut virus (IRKV). Bokeloh bat lyssavirus also appears to belong to this group (CFSPH 2012). Lagos bat virus (LBV), Mokola virus (MOKV), and Shimoni bat virus (SHIBV) belong to Phylogroup 2. West Caucasian bat virus (WCBV) does not cross-react serologically with any of the two phylogroups and has been provisionally placed in a new group, Phylogroup III (Rabies Bulletin Europe 2012; CFSPH 2012). There is a significant serological neutralisation within phylogroups, but very limited cross-neutralisation has been detected between phylogroups.

The classical rabies virus is found worldwide and is the causative agent of classical rabies. It is responsible for the overwhelming majority of reported rabies cases in animals and humans. Other lyssaviruses appear to have more restricted geographical and host range, with the majority having been isolated from bats; however, it can be assumed that all lyssaviruses can cause indistinguishable fatal encephalitis both in humans and in other mammals (OIE Terrestrial Manual 2011; Rabies Bulletin Europe 2012).

Rhabdoviruses are approximately 180 nm long and 75 nm wide. The RNA genome of lyssaviruses is 12 kilobases long, non-segmented, and of negative polarity encoding five viral proteins: nucleoprotein (N), phosphoprotein (P), matrix protein (M), glycoprotein (G), and polymerase (L). There is a leader sequence (LDR) of approximately 50 nucleotides, followed by N, P, M, G, and L genes (CDC 2012b; WHO 2012; Rabies Bulletin Europe 2012). All rhabdoviruses have two major structural components: a helical ribonucleoprotein core (RNP) and a surrounding envelope. In the RNP, genomic RNA is tightly encased by the nucleoprotein. Two other viral proteins, the phosphoprotein and the large protein (L protein or polymerase), are associated with the RNP. The glycoprotein forms

Table 2.1 Taxonomy of lyssaviruses (ICTV 2012; Rabies Bulletin Europe 2012)

Species	Potential vector(s)/reservoirs	Distribution
Rabies virus-type species	Carnivores (worldwide), bats (Americas)	Worldwide (except several islands)
Aravan virus	Insectivorous bats (*Myotis blythi*)	Central Asia
Australian bat lyssavirus	Frugivorous/insectivorous bats (*Megachiroptera/Microchiroptera*)	Australia
Duvenhage virus	Insectivorous bats	Southern Africa
European bat lyssavirus 1	Insectivorous bats (*Eptesicus serotinus*)	Europe
European bat lyssavirus 2	Insectivorous bats (*Myotis daubentonii, M. dasycneme*)	Europe
Irkut virus	Insectivorous bats (*Murina leucogaster*)	East Siberia
Khujand virus	Insectivorous bats (*Myotis mystacinus*)	Central Asia
Lagos bat virus	Frugivorous bats (*Megachiroptera*)	Africa
Mokola virus	?	Sub-Saharan Africa
Shimoni bat virus	Commerson's leaf-nosed bat (*Hipposideros commersoni*)	East Africa
West Caucasian bat virus	Insectivorous bats (*Miniopterus schreibersi*)	Caucasian region

Fig. 2.2 General structure of a rhabdovirus (Hunt 2012)

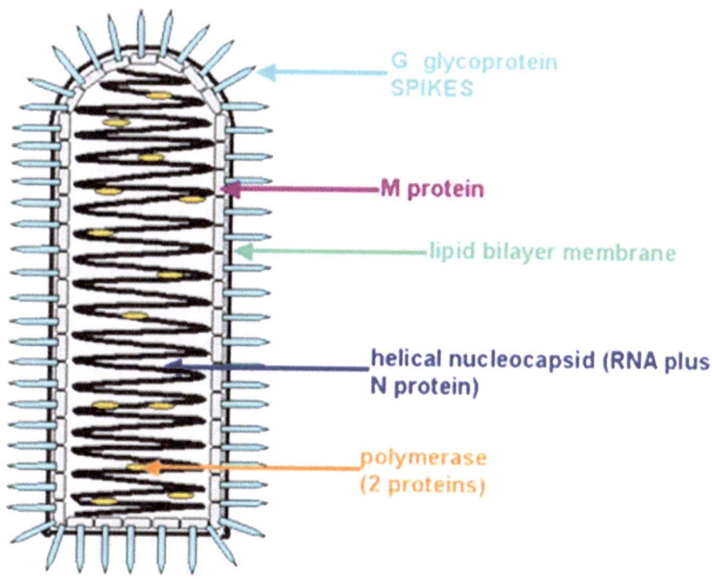

approximately 400 trimeric spikes which are tightly arranged on the surface of the virus. The M protein is associated with both the envelope and the RNP and may be the central protein of rhabdovirus assembly (Fig. 2.2).

2.2 Mode of Transmission

All species of mammals are susceptible to rabies virus infection, but only a few species are important as reservoirs for the disease. The virus is readily transmitted between mammals, whether they are the same or different species. It is usually transmitted through saliva when infected saliva of a host is passed to an uninfected animal. As rabid animals become aggressive and harbour the virus in saliva, the transmission of virus is frequently via animal bites. Less often, an animal or person is infected by contact with infectious saliva or neurological tissues, through mucous membrane or abraded skin, for example, when the infected material gets directly into the eyes, nose, mouth, or a wound. Licking of abraded or broken skin by

Fig. 2.3 Rabies transmission pathways

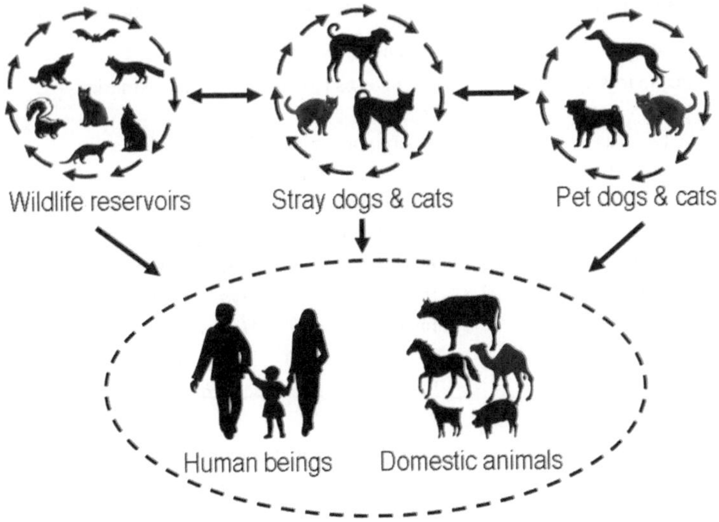

an infected animal may cause infection but rabies virus is not transmitted through intact skin. Scratches, abrasions, open wounds, or mucous membranes getting contaminated with saliva or other potentially infectious material constitute non-bite exposures (CDC 2012b).

Dogs are the main hosts that are responsible for most of the human cases in Asia and Africa. In the developed countries in Europe, North America, and Australia, rabies is present mainly in the wildlife hosts, from which the disease spills over to domestic animals and humans. The bite of infected dogs, cats, and wild carnivorous animals including vampire bats is the most frequent way of transmission of rabies infection to humans. Cattle, horses, deer, and other herbivorous animals can become infected and can be potential source of transmission of the virus, but it is not common (Fig. 2.3).

Inhalation of aerosolised rabies virus is another potential non-bite route of exposure (CDC 2012a). Aerosol transmission has been documented in laboratories and bat caves. Rabies viruses have been transmitted by ingestion in experimentally infected animals, and there is anecdotal evidence of transmission in milk to a lamb and a human infant from their mothers (CFSPH 2012).

Rabies virus is killed by heating; therefore consuming pasteurised milk or cooked meat is not an exposure. However, drinking unpasteurised milk from a rabid cow/goat is considered an exposure (Partners for Rabies Prevention 2010). In two incidents investigated by the US Centers for Disease Control and Prevention (CDC), people who drank unpasteurised milk from rabid cows were given postexposure prophylaxis (PEP) against rabies (CFSPH 2012).

There are few well-documented cases of human-to-human transmission of rabies through corneal transplants and recently through solid organ (pancreas, kidney, liver) transplants. In addition to this, bite and non-bite exposures inflicted by infected humans could theoretically transmit rabies, but no such cases have been documented. Casual contact, such as touching a person with rabies or contact with non-infectious fluid or tissue (urine, blood, faeces) does not constitute an exposure (CDC 2012a).

2.3 Pathogenesis

Immediately after infection through cut, broken, or abraded skin or through mucous membrane, the rabies virus enters an eclipse phase during which it is not easily detected. During this phase, initial virus multiplication occurs in non-nervous tissue such as striated muscle cells at the site (Radostits et al. 2007). Here the virus can remain

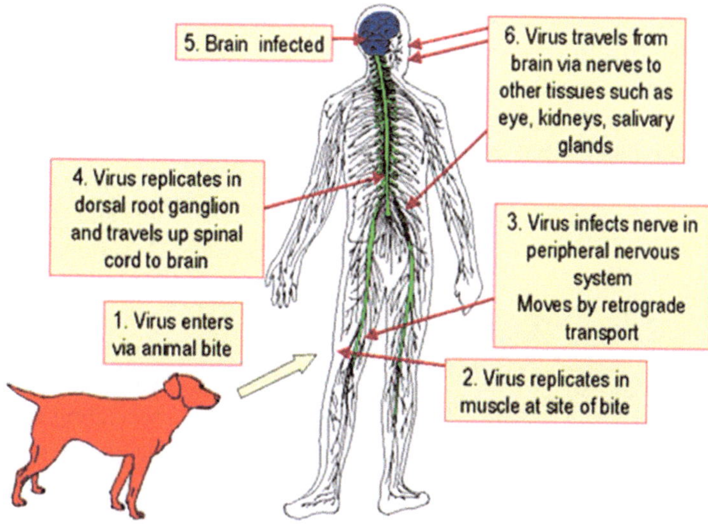

Fig. 2.4 Progression of rabies virus infection in body (Hunt 2012)

for a prolonged period of time which influences the incubation period (time between the exposure and onset of disease) in individual cases. The virus binds to the cells at the site of the inoculation via nicotinic acetylcholine receptors. The replication in muscle cells occurs with no obvious symptoms (Hunt 2012). It does not usually stimulate an immune response at this time, but it is susceptible to neutralisation if antibodies are present (Fig. 2.4).

The virus being neurotropic, its uptake into the peripheral nerves is important for progressive infection. The neuromuscular spindles provide an important site of virus entry into the nervous system. Entry into the nervous system may also occur at motor end plates (Radostits et al. 2007). After the entry of the virus into a nerve, there is invasion of the brain by passive movement of the virus within axons, first into the spinal cord and then into the brain. This method of spread accounts for the extreme variations in the incubation period in different cases depending upon the site of the bite (proximity to the brain). Bites on the head usually result in a shorter incubation period than bites on the extremities. The whole process of infection and its progression is divided into the following stages (CDC 2012b):

1. Adsorption (receptors and virion interaction)
2. Penetration (virus entry)
3. Uncoating (envelope removal)
4. Transcription (synthesis of mRNAs)
5. Translation (synthesis of structural proteins)
6. Processing (G-protein glycosylation)
7. Replication (production of genomic RNA from intermediate strand)
8. Assembly
9. Budding (complete virions)

Adsorption involves fusion of the rabies virus envelope to the host cell membrane in which interaction of the G protein and specific cell surface receptors may be involved. Adsorption initiates the infection process, after which the virus penetrates the host cell and enters the cytoplasm by pinocytosis (via clathrin-coated pits). The virions aggregate in the large endosomes (cytoplasmic vesicles) and the viral membranes fuse to the endosomal membranes. It results in uncoating due to the release of viral RNP into the cytoplasm. Transcription of messenger RNAs (mRNAs) then takes place to permit virus replication (CDC 2012b).

A viral-encoded polymerase (L gene) transcribes the genomic strand of rabies RNA into leader RNA and five capped and polyadenylated mRNAs, which are translated into N, P, M, G, and L proteins. The intracellular ratio of leader RNA to N protein regulates the beginning of the replication process. It begins with the synthesis of full-length copies (positive strands) of the viral genome that serve as templates for synthesis of full-length negative strands of the viral genome (CDC 2012b).

Virus replication is followed by the assembly process and budding. The N–P–L complex encapsulates the negative-stranded genomic RNA to form the RNP core, and the M protein forms a capsule, or matrix, around the RNP. The M–RNP complex binds with the glycoprotein in the plasma membrane, and the completed virus buds from it (CDC 2012b).

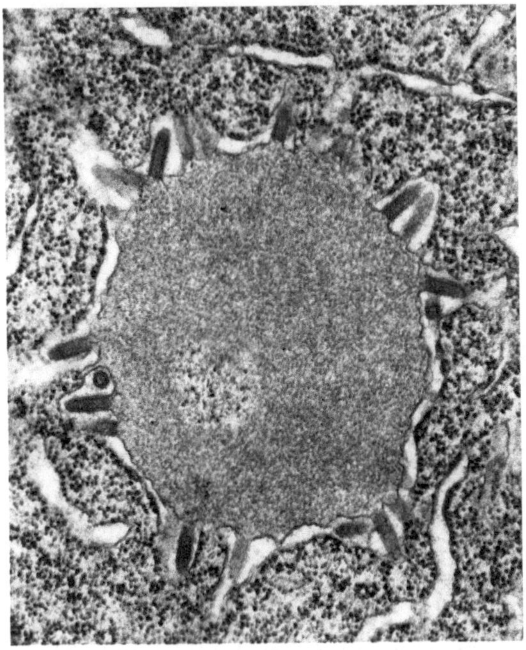

Fig. 2.5 Rabies virus infection in hamster brain, showing an early stage in the formation of a Negri body and some virions budding from intracytoplasmic membranes surrounding the Negri body. Magnification approximately ×30,000 (Murphy 2012)

The virus moves along the nerve axons to the central nervous system (CNS) using retrograde transport. The virus arrives at the dorsal root ganglia and spinal cord and then spreads to the brain. A variety of cells in the brain can be infected including in the cerebellum, the Purkinje's cells, and also cells of the hippocampus and pontine nuclei (Hunt 2012). Following the entry of rabies virus to the CNS, usually in the spinal cord, an ascending wave of neuronal infection and neuronal dysfunction occurs.

After the virus has multiplied in the brain causing inflammation, almost all animals begin to show the first signs of rabies (prodromal phase). The primary lesions produced are in the CNS (Figs. 2.5 and 2.6), and the spread from the site of infection occurs only by way of the peripheral nerves. The virus moves from the brain to the salivary glands and saliva (Fig. 2.7). Within the CNS, there is preferential viral budding from plasma membranes. Conversely, virus in the salivary glands buds primarily from the cell membrane into the acinar lumen.

Within a short period of time (usually 3–5 days), the virus causes enough damage to the brain and the signs of rabies become more clear and peculiar (CDC 2012b). During this neurological phase, the virus is distributed to highly innervated tissues via the peripheral nerves. The virus can spread from the CNS, via neurons, to

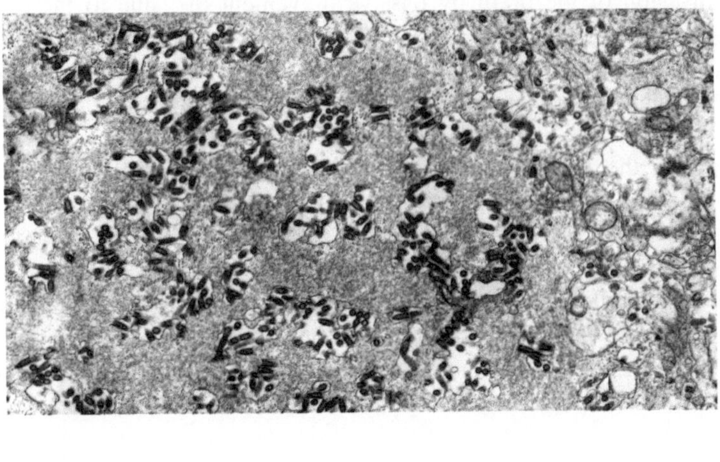

Fig. 2.6 Rabies virus infection in hamster brain, showing large numbers of *bullet-shaped* virions in the cytoplasm of an infected neuron. Magnification approximately ×25,000 (Murphy 2012)

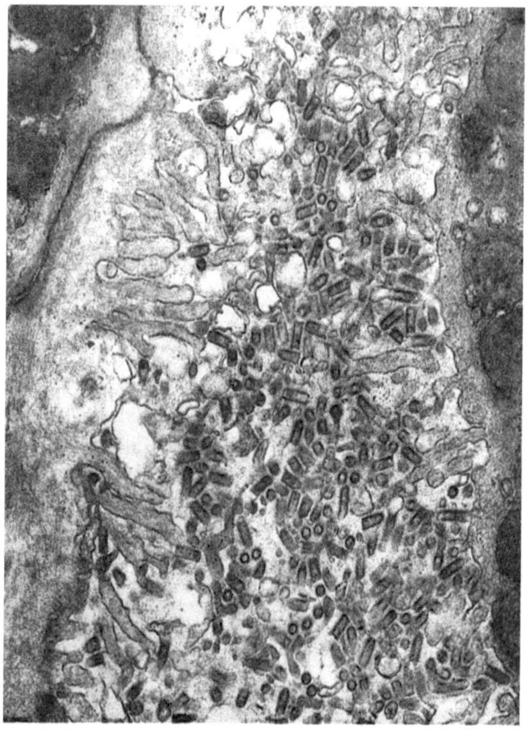

Fig. 2.7 Rabies virus in the salivary gland of a rabid fox. Magnification approximately ×40,000 (Murphy 2012)

the skin, eye, and various other sites. Infection of the brain leads to encephalitis and neural degeneration although elsewhere the virus seems to cause little in the way of a cytopathic effect. Gradually ascending paralysis of the hindquarters may be followed by severe signs of mania, which persist almost until death. Destruction of spinal neurons results in paralysis, but when the virus invades the brain, irritation of higher centres produces manias, excitement, and convulsions. The clinical signs of salivation, indigestion and pica, paralysis of bladder and anus, and increased libido all suggest involvement of the autonomic nervous system, including endocrine glands. Death is usually due to respiratory paralysis (Radostits et al. 2007; Hunt 2012).

Studies have shown that rabies virus can be excreted in the saliva of infected animals several days before the illness is apparent. Wildlife species are also known to excrete rabies virus in saliva before the onset of signs of illness. The excretion of virus may be intermittent, and the relative amount of excreted virus may vary greatly over time, before and after the onset of clinical signs (CDC 2012b).

Many factors influence the incubation period including the site of the exposure (proximity of the site of infection to the brain), type of rabies virus, number of virus particles in the infection, and the immunological status of the exposed animal or person.

The immune response to the naturally acquired virus is slow and a good neutralising response is not seen until the virus has reached the brain which is too late for survival. Neutralising antibody and inflammatory infiltration are usually absent at the time of onset of encephalitic signs. Antibody titres reach substantial levels only in the terminal stages of the disease. Cell-mediated immunity plays little role in a rabies infection. Rabies is almost always fatal and only very few survivors of symptomatic rabies have been documented (Hunt 2012; CDC 2012a).

2.4 Predisposing and Risk Factors

Continual, frequent, or increased chance of exposure to the rabies virus predisposes a person to greater risk of infection. Certain categories of people fall in the high-risk group as a result of either their place of residence or their occupation. For example, the people living in developing countries or travelling to the rabies-endemic areas, including countries in Africa and Southeast Asia, may suffer more. Similarly, the activities that involve frequent contact with animals or exposure to animal bites also heighten the risk of exposure. Veterinarians, animal handlers, animal control officers, dogcatchers, quarantine officers, pet owners, schoolchildren, postmen, delivery personnel, etc. fall in this category.

Handling of rabies virus and other lyssaviruses and infected animals may expose the laboratory workers to rabies infection. Wildlife wardens and others who come in frequent contact with wild animals are also at greater risk. The people engaged in exploring caves infested with bats or those camping in forests without taking precautions to keep wild animals and bats away may also expose themselves to rabies.

Besides the concentration of virus entering the bite wounds, the closeness of bite wound to the head or neck increases the chances of disease as the rabies virus travels more quickly to the brain.

The unavailability of adequate medical facilities, vaccines, and immunoglobulin in rural high-risk areas makes the residents and travellers more vulnerable to the disease.

Clearing of forests and disturbed wildlife habitats may lead to straying of wild animals into the nearby areas resulting in spillover of the infection to domestic or pet animals as well as to human beings. The risk factors that may expose pets to rabies infection include exposure to wildlife, exposure to other unvaccinated pets, and exposure to stray unvaccinated animals.

References

Blancou J (2004) Rabies in Europe and the Mediterranean basin: from antiquity to the 19th century. In: King AA, Fooks AR, Aubert M, Wandeler AI (eds) Historical perspective of rabies in Europe and the Mediterranean basin. World Organisation for Animal Health, Paris, pp 15–24

CDC (2012a) Rabies. Centers for Disease Control and Prevention. http://www.cdc.gov/rabies/. Accessed 30 Mar 2012

CDC (2012b) The rabies virus. Centers for Disease Control and Prevention. http://www.cdc.gov/rabies/transmission/virus.html. Accessed 30 Mar 2012

CFSPH (2012) Rabies. The Center for Food Security and Public Health, Iowa State University, Iowa State University. Iowa. http://www.cfsph.iastate.edu/Factsheets/pdfs/rabies.pdf. Accessed 9 June 2013

Freuling CM, Beer M, Conraths FJ, Finke S, Hoffmann B, Keller B, Kliemt J, Mettenleiter TC, Mühlbach E, Teifke JP, Wohlsein P, Müller T (2011) Novel lyssavirus in Natterer's bat, Germany. Emerg Infect Dis 17:1519–1522

Hunt R (2012) Rabies. Microbiology and Immunology On-line, University of South Carolina School of Medicine. http://www.microbiologybook.org/virol/rabies.htm. Accessed 17 Aug 2012

ICTV (2012) Virus taxonomy: 2012 release. International Committee on Taxonomy of Viruses. http://www.ictvonline.org. Accessed 9 June 2013

Marston DA, Horton DL, Ngeleja C, Hampson K, McElhinney LM, Banyard AC, Haydon D, Cleaveland S, Rupprecht CE, Bigambo M, Fooks AR, Lembo T (2012) Ikoma lyssavirus, highly divergent novel lyssavirus in an African civet. Emerg Infect Dis 18:664–667

Murphy FA (2012). Virus images/Foundations of virology. The University of Texas Medical Branch at Galveston, Department of Pathology, Galveston, TX 77555–0609 USA. http://www.utmb.edu/virusimages/. Accessed 17 Aug 2012

Mutinelli F, Stankov S, Hristovski M, Seimenis A, Theoharakou H, Vodopija I (2004) Rabies in Italy, Yugoslavia, Croatia, Bosnia, Slovenia, Macedonia, Albania & Greece. In: King AA, Fooks AR, Aubert M, Wandeler AI (eds) Historical perspective of rabies in Europe and the Mediterranean basin. World Organisation for Animal Health, Paris, pp 93–118

OIE Terrestrial Manual (2011) Manual of diagnostic tests and vaccines for terrestrial animals 2011. Chapter 2.1.13. Rabies. World Organisation for Animal Health, http://www.oie.int/international-standard-setting/terrestrial-manual/access-online/. Accessed 31 Mar 2012

Partners for Rabies Prevention (2010) Blueprint for rabies prevention and control. http://www.rabiesblueprint.com/. Accessed 12 Apr 2012

Rabies Bulletin Europe (2012) Rabies Information System of the WHO Collaboration Centre for Rabies Surveillance and Research. http://www.who-rabies-bulletin.org. Accessed 8 Apr 2012

Radostits OM, Gay CC, Hinchcliff KW, Constable PD (2007) Veterinary medicine: a textbook of the diseases of cattle, horses, sheep, pigs and goats, 10th edn. Saunders-Elsevier, Edinburgh

Smithcors JF (1958) The history of some current problems in animal disease. VII. Rabies (Part I). Vet Med 53:149–154

Théodoridès J (1986) Histoire de la rage. Cave Canem. Fondation Singer Polignac Masson, Paris, 289 pp

WHO (2012) Rabies. World Health Organization. www.who.int. Accessed 10 Mar 2012

3 Epidemiology

Abstract

Rabies is widely distributed with the exception of only a few countries. People of all age groups are susceptible but children are at a greater risk. Rabies is maintained in two epidemiological cycles, urban cycle and sylvatic cycle. Dogs are the main reservoir hosts in the urban cycle which predominates in India and many other developing countries in Asia, Africa, and Central and South America. Sylvatic cycle is predominant in Europe and North America because of successful control of dog rabies. In some regions including India, sylvatic cycle operates simultaneously with the urban cycle, making the epidemiology of rabies more complex. The maximum burden of rabies lies in Asia followed by Africa, while rabies is endemic in animal populations in many European countries. In Latin America, rabies circulates in dogs and bats. Bats are the source of most human rabies cases in the USA and Canada. Bats in Australia have been found to carry Australian bat lyssavirus. A variety of bat lyssaviruses have also been documented in Africa. Due to the recent reports of Asian bats maintaining lyssaviruses, interest in the role of bats in rabies transmission has increased in Asia.

3.1 Epidemiological Features

Rabies is widely distributed across the globe, with only a few countries (mainly islands and peninsulas) being free of the disease. The disease occurs in more than 150 countries and territories. Worldwide, more than 55,000 people die of rabies every year. Although all age groups are susceptible, children are at a greater risk. Forty per cent of people who are bitten by suspect rabid animals are children under 15 years of age, and the majority receiving treatment are males (WHO 2012).

Rabies is maintained in two epidemiological cycles, urban cycle and sylvatic cycle. In the urban rabies cycle, dogs are the main reservoir host. This cycle predominates in India and many other developing countries in Africa, Asia, and Central and South America with large populations of stray and unvaccinated dogs. Less-industrialised countries, especially where there is a large population of ownerless dogs, face greater risk of dog rabies. Overall, dogs are the source of 99 % of human rabies deaths. Dog rabies potentially threatens over 3.3 billion people in Africa and Asia (WHO 2012).

S.R. Garg, *Rabies in Man and Animals*, DOI 10.1007/978-81-322-1605-6_3,

Dog rabies transmission cycle has been virtually eliminated in North America and Europe, although sporadic cases occur in dogs infected by wild animals. Due to strict surveillance and control measures in these countries, the urban cycle is not perpetuated in the dog population usually. However, wildlife reservoirs have become increasingly important in rabies transmission in such areas (WHO 2012). The sylvatic (or wildlife) cycle is, therefore, the predominant cycle in Europe and North America. This type of transmission cycle involves one or more carnivorous wildlife species. For example, in Europe, the red fox (*Vulpes vulpes*) is the main reservoir species. In parts of Asia, the raccoon dog (*Nyctereutes procyonoides*) is also considered reservoir species for rabies. The introduced raccoon dogs in Eastern Europe may also be implicated in sustaining the chain of infection. In the Americas, bat species are additional reservoir for rabies virus (Rabies Bulletin Europe 2012). However, different infection cycles may occur simultaneously within one geographical region. For example, independent rabies infectious cycles in raccoons (*Procyon lotor*), skunks (*Mephitis* sp.), red foxes (*Vulpes vulpes*), grey foxes (*Urocyon cinereoargenteus*), coyotes (*Canis latrans*), and arctic foxes (*Alopex lagopus*) exist in the Americas. Wildlife rabies is sporadically transmitted to domestic animals and to humans (Rabies Bulletin Europe 2012).

More dangerously, in some parts of the world, the sylvatic cycle operates simultaneously with the urban cycle, making the rabies epidemiology more complex. In India, disease transmission is known to involve domestic animals (urban cycle) as well as wild animals (sylvatic cycle), the former being a more common source. Wild animals in India are rarely implicated in the spread of disease to man. People most at risk live in rural areas where human vaccines and immunoglobulin are not readily available or accessible (WHO 2012). Poor people are at a greater risk, as the average cost of rabies postexposure prophylaxis (PEP) after contact with a suspected rabid animal is US$40 in Africa and US$49 in Asia, while the average daily income per person is very low (WHO 2012).

Depending on the rabies risks in terrestrial animals, the Health Protection Agency (2012) of UK and the Health Protection Scotland (2012) divide different countries into three categories: (1) those with 'no risk' of rabies, (2) those with 'low risk' of rabies, and (3) those with 'high risk' of rabies (Table 3.1).

3.2 Rabies in Asia

Asia bears the maximum burden of rabies. According to the WHO estimates, 31,000 human rabies deaths occur annually in Asia which comes to about 56 % of total global deaths due to rabies. As most of the developing countries in Asia have weak surveillance and reporting systems, the true number of fatalities can be even higher.

The main route of transmission is through the bites of rabid dogs. More than three billion people in the developing countries in Asia are potentially exposed to dog rabies (WHO Global Vaccine Research Forum 2006). Human cases have also been reported due to exposure to rabid cats and wildlife. Mongoose, jackals, foxes, and wolves have been incriminated as wildlife reservoirs of rabies (Gongal and Wright 2011). The categorisation of Asian and the Middle East countries according to the rabies risks in terrestrial animals has been shown in Table 3.1.

More than 1.4 billion people are at potential risk of rabies infection in the Southeast Asian region. The estimated number of dog bites in human beings in the region is about 19 million while 21,000–24,000 people die due to rabies each year. This accounts for about 45 % of the worldwide human rabies deaths (Gongal and Wright 2011).

In a survey conducted in the year 2003, the annual incidence of human deaths due to rabies in India was estimated at 20,565, which is about 2 per 100,000 population (Sudarshan et al. 2007). The majority victims were male, adult, from rural areas, and unvaccinated persons. The study revealed dogs to be responsible for 96.2 % human rabies deaths while cats and other animals accounted for 1.7 % and 2.1 % cases, respectively. Two deaths due to the bites from jackals were also recorded. Among the dogs, 75.2 % were stray dogs.

Table 3.1 Rabies risk in different countries (updated to 12 March 2012)[1] (Health Protection Scotland 2012; Health Protection Agency 2012)

Risk of rabies by country	Region	Countries	Comments
'No risk' of rabies Animals originating from these countries and territories are considered to pose 'no risk' of rabies (free of terrestrial rabies)	Africa	Ascension Island, Madeira, Mauritius, Seychelles, St. Helena, Reunion	–
	Americas	Anguilla, Antigua and Barbuda, Aruba, Bahamas, Barbados, Bermuda, Cayman Islands, Dominica, Easter Island, Falklands, Galapagos Islands, Guadeloupe, Hawaii, Jamaica, Martinique, Montserrat, Netherlands Antilles, South Georgia and South Sandwich Islands, St. Kitts and Nevis, St. Lucia, St Pierre and Miquelon, St. Vincent and the Grenadines, Tahiti, Turks and Caicos Islands, Virgin Islands	–
	Antarctica	Antarctica	–
	Asia	Japan, Singapore, Taiwan	–
	Europe	Andorra, Austria, Azores, Belgium, Cyprus, Czech Republic, Denmark, Faroe Islands, Finland, France (including Corsica), Germany, Gibraltar, Greece, Iceland, Ireland, Liechtenstein, Luxembourg, Malta, Monaco, The Netherlands, Norway, Portugal, San Marino, Spain, Sweden, Switzerland, UK	Italy – 20 cases in wild animals in 2009 Northeast Italy Belgium – no cases in 2009 Finland – one bat case in 2009 Spain – mainland and islands rabies free
	Oceania	Australia, Christmas Island, Cocos (Keeling) Island, Cook Island, French Polynesia, Guam, New Caledonia, New Zealand, Norfolk Islands, Northern Mariana Islands, Palau, Pitcairn Island, Tokelau, Wake Island, Wallis and Futuna Islands	–
'Low risk' of rabies Animals originating from these countries are considered to pose a 'low risk' of rabies	Americas	Canada, French Guiana, Grenada, Trinidad and Tobago, USA, Uruguay	USA (CDC, Atlanta [http://www.cdc.gov/] provides information on the risk of rabies in different parts of the USA)
	Asia and the Middle East	Bahrain, Brunei Darussalam, Hong Kong (China), Kuwait, the Maldives, Qatar, United Arab Emirates	–
	Europe	Bulgaria[a], Italy[a] (northern and eastern border regions only), Jan Mayen and Svalbard (Norway)	[a]Bulgaria – 10 cases reported in domestic animals and 48 cases reported in nondomestic animals 2009 [a]Italy – 20 cases in wild animals in 2009
	Oceania	American Samoa, Fiji, Kiribati, Marshall Islands, Micronesia, Nauru, Niue, Papua New Guinea, Samoa, Sao Tome and Principe, Solomon Islands, Tonga, Tuvalu, Vanuatu	–

(continued)

Table 3.1 (continued)

Risk of rabies by country	Region	Countries	Comments
'High risk' of rabies Animals originating from countries where terrestrial rabies is enzootic are considered 'high risk'	Africa	Algeria, Angola, Benin, Botswana, Burkina Faso, Burundi, Cape Verde, Central African Republic, Chad, Comoros, Congo, Congo (DRC), Ceuta and Melilla (autonomous Spanish cities in N. Africa), Djibouti, Egypt, Equatorial Guinea, Eritrea, Ethiopia, Gabon, Gambia, Ghana, Guinea, Guinea- Bissau, Ivory Coast, Kenya, Lesotho, Liberia, Libya, Madagascar, Malawi, Mali, Mauritania, Mayotte, Morocco, Mozambique, Namibia, Niger, Nigeria, Rwanda, Senegal, Sierra Leone, Somalia, South Africa, South Sudan, Sudan, Swaziland, Tanzania (including Zanzibar), Togo, Tunisia, Uganda, Zambia, Zimbabwe	–
	Americas	Argentina, Belize, Bolivia, Brazil, Chile, Colombia, Costa Rica, Cuba, Dominican Republic, Ecuador, El Salvador, Guatemala, Guyana, Haiti, Honduras, Mexico, Nicaragua, Panama, Paraguay, Peru, Puerto Rico, Suriname, Venezuela (including Margarita island)	–
	Asia	Afghanistan, Bangladesh, Bhutan, Borneo, Cambodia, China (including Macau), East Timor, India (including Andaman and Nicobar islands), Indonesia, Kazakhstan, Korea (N), Korea (S), Kyrgyzstan, Laos, Malaysia, Mongolia, Myanmar, Nepal, Pakistan, Philippines, Sri Lanka, Tajikistan, Thailand, Turkmenistan, Uzbekistan, Vietnam	–
	Europe	Albania, Armenia, Azerbaijan, Belarus, Bosnia and Herzegovina, Hungary, Croatia, Estonia, Georgia, Greenland, Kosovo, Latvia, Lithuania, Macedonia, Moldova, Montenegro, Poland, Romania, Russia, Serbia, Slovakia, Slovenia, Turkey, Ukraine	–
	The Middle East	Iran, Iraq, Israel, Jordan, Lebanon, Oman, Saudi Arabia, Syria, Yemen	–
Countries (and islands) not otherwise mentioned as 'no risk' or 'low risk' should be considered as 'high risk'			

[1] Adapted by the Health Protection Scotland (2012) from Health Protection Agency – Rabies Risks by Country [http://www.hpa.org.uk/web/HPAweb&HPAwebStandard/HPAweb_C/1259152458758#S]

[a] Most recent cases information obtained from WHO Rabies Bulletin Europe [http://www.who-rabies-bulletin.org]

Notes: A country may be considered free from classical rabies when all the following apply:

- Rabies in animals is notifiable
- An effective system of disease surveillance in animals is in operation
- All regulatory measures for the prevention and control of rabies in animals have been implemented, including effective importation procedures
- No case of indigenously acquired classical rabies infection has been confirmed in man or any animal species during the previous 2 years (this status would not be affected by the isolation of a bat lyssavirus such as European bat lyssavirus 1 or 2)
- No imported case in carnivores has been confirmed outside a quarantine station for the previous 6 months

In Pakistan, although there are no accurate data, it is estimated that over 25,000 animal bites and 2,000–5,000 rabies deaths occur a year. Over 90 % animal bites are from dogs, other animals being cats, cattle, and wolves. Most bites occur in rural areas; however, majority of victims do not seek medical attention and depend on home remedies alone (Salahuddin 2009). In Bangladesh, the annual estimated number of human rabies death is 10,000, though few records frequently underrate the figure. Annual number of animal bite exposures in Bangladesh is estimated to be more than 100,000. About 95 % of the reservoir animals of rabies are stray dogs, while cat, jackal, mongoose, etc. cover the remaining (Rahman 2009).

In Nepal, most (94 %) of the human rabies cases follow contacts with rabid dogs. It is estimated that on an average 200 people die annually due to rabies. National statistics shows that about 30,000 people receive PEP and about 55,000 dogs are immunised against rabies with a tissue culture vaccine produced in the country. An epidemiological surveillance was carried out during the years 2005–2007. Suspected rabid dog bite human cases were 16,812, 16,401, and 20,943 for the year 2005, 2006, and 2007, respectively, while the human mortality due to rabies was 1.5 %, 1.4 %, and 2.17 %, respectively (Joshi 2009). In Bhutan, there were 753 cases of rabies reported in domestic animal species from January 1998 to March 2006 (Rinzin 2009).

In Sri Lanka, dog is the main reservoir of rabies and the estimated dog population is 2.5 million. A community survey conducted in 1997 revealed that the incidence of dog bites was 13.2 per 1,000 population (1.3 %). Another study showed that 7.55 per 1,000 (0.75 %) population had taken postexposure treatment in the year 2003. In the year 2008, an estimated number of 174,000 animal bite victims were initiated with rabies PEP at government hospitals (Harischandra 2009a, b).

In the Philippines, rabies is responsible for death of 200–300 Filipinos annually. In 2008, 250 human rabies cases were reported in the country. Majority of these persons were males and at least a third of them were less than 15 years of age. About 190,000 animal bites were reported. Canine rabies is endemic in the country, and the exposure through animal bites is responsible for almost all human rabies in the Philippines. Animal rabies is prevalent in almost all parts of the country except in some island provinces and municipalities. Rabies among animals has been limited to domesticated animals. In 2008, 971 animal rabies cases were reported, 98 % of which were dogs (Deray 2009).

Rabies situation in Thailand has been improving both in animals and humans during the past decade. The human fatality due to rabies declined from 57 in 1998 to 9 in 2008. The number of animal bites or exposures per year varies from 300,000 to 400,000 (Panichabhongse 2009). In Vietnam, dogs and cats are main rabies reservoir. Among those who received postexposure treatment, the exposure was through the dog bites in 86.6 % persons and through cat bites in 8 % cases. The rabies fatality rate was 0.107 per 100,000 population in 2008 (Hien 2009).

In Cambodia, 124,749 patients received PEP during 1998–2007 at Institut Pasteur (average 12,470; range 8,907–14,475) and 63 fatal human cases presented with encephalitis following a dog bite were reported. During this period, out of 1,255 animal brain samples examined, 97 % were from dogs that included 610 (49 %) positive samples (Vong 2009).

Human rabies cases showed an increasing trend in China in the recent past and reached the highest peak in 2007. The human rabies cases reported in the country between 1996 and 2008 predominately occurred in the rural areas and mainly involved the peasants, students, and unattended children. Among these, 85–95 % cases were exposed to dogs and 4–10 % to cats. Reports of human rabies cases exposed to wild animals showed an increase in recent years (Tang 2009).

Most part of the territories of Mongolia has active rabies natural foci. Thirty-four reports of human rabies cases were recorded during 1996–2008 in the country. Among these, 20 (58.8 %) were males and 14 (41.2 %) were females. Children in the age group 0–9 years were the most affected (41.2 %). Dogs, wolves, and foxes play main role in the rabies cycle. About 49 % of all the people exposed to animal bites were bitten by dogs, 35 % by wolves, 2 % by foxes, and 14 % by livestock. Apart from human cases, 1,535 cases of animal rabies were recorded during the same period, 82 % of which were livestock and 15.3 % dogs (Undraa 2009).

Japan has been free of rabies for more than past half century. The last cases of indigenous human and animal rabies were in 1954 and 1957, respectively. In 1970, a college student suffered from rabies in Tokyo after a trip to Nepal where he had been bitten by a stray dog. In November 2006, two patients with a history of dog bites in the Philippines were suspected of rabies. Phylogenetic analysis of the amplified viral gene demonstrated that both isolates were closely related to canine rabies variants circulating in the Philippines (Inoue 2009).

The incidence of rabies in animals reported to the OIE by different Asian countries during the period 2005–2011 (OIE 2013) has been presented in Table 3.2.

3.3 Rabies in Africa

Africa is the second most rabies-affected continent after Asia. Most of the countries in Africa present high risk of rabies (Table 3.1). The estimate of annual human rabies deaths in the continent is 24,000, about 4 per 100,000 population at risk (WHO 2012). Thus, 44 % of the estimated human deaths due to rabies worldwide occur in Africa; however, the mortality figure is still considered to be a conservative estimate as rabies cases in humans are widely under-reported in parts of Africa (Cleaveland et al. 2002; Mallewa et al. 2007). Rabies virus is enzootic throughout Africa with the domestic dog (*Canis familiaris*) as the principal vector (Knobel et al. 2005). Sylvatic rabies is also reported in a number of wildlife hosts, particularly in southern Africa (Nel et al. 1993; Swanepoel et al. 1993; von Teichman et al. 1995; Knobel et al. 2005; Davis et al. 2007).

The first confirmed outbreak of rabies in Africa, believed to have followed the importation of an infected dog from England in 1892, occurred in the Eastern Cape Province of South Africa (Swanepoel et al. 1993). In a recent study, the evolutionary dynamics of rabies virus in western and central Africa was investigated by sequencing 92 isolates sampled from 27 African countries over 29 years. The study revealed that rabies virus currently circulating in dogs in that region fell into a single lineage designated Africa 2, and the analysis of phylogeographical structure revealed its possible east-to-west spread across Africa (Talbi et al. 2009). In addition, the study suggested that the Africa 2 lineage was introduced into the region probably <200 years ago. The emergence and dissemination of the rabies virus thus coincided with the expanding European colonisation and urbanisation, perhaps occupying the entire region in a 100 year period.

From about 1947 onwards, an invasive form of dog rabies spread in different parts of the continent which was followed by the emergence of rabies in jackals and cattle. The existence of endemic rabies of viverrids (mongooses and genets) was confirmed in South Africa in 1928, and since then, the viverrid disease has continued to occur widely with spillover of infection to cattle and a variety of other animals. The cases of rabies in kudu antelope and bat-eared fox have been recognised. The rabies-related viruses, Lagos bat, Mokola, and Duvenhage, associated with bats, shrews, and rodents in Africa, are also known to have caused disease (Swanepoel et al. 1993).

A number of African countries have been reporting the incidence of rabies in animals to OIE. Country-wise reported incidence of animal rabies during the period 2005–2011 (OIE 2013) is shown in Table 3.3.

3.4 Rabies in Europe

Rabies remains endemic in animal populations in many European countries, especially in Central and Eastern Europe despite systematic efforts for rabies control, surveillance, and monitoring of rabies by international organisations. The situation in different countries however greatly varies (Table 3.1). The principal reservoirs of classical rabies in Europe are red foxes (*Vulpes vulpes*)

Table 3.2 Incidence of rabies in animals in Asian countries (2005–2011) (OIE 2013)

	New outbreaks[a]						
Country	2005	2006	2007	2008	2009	2010	2011
Afghanistan	+..	…	…	…	?	4	7
Bahrain	0	0	0	0	0	0	0
Bangladesh	…	…	+..	+..	+..	+..	+..
Bhutan	15	12	6	23	10	11	4
Brunei Darussalam	0	0	0	0	0	0	0
Cambodia	…	…	…	…	…	0	?
China (People's Rep. of)	145	90	72	33	26	21	20
Chinese Taipei	0	0	0	0	0	0	0
Hong Kong (SAR-PRC)	…	…	…	0	0	0	o
India	31	17	43	47	97	71	92
Indonesia	+()	+()	+	+	+	+	+
Iran	297	370	150	419	200	130	187
Iraq	…	…	+()	+()	…	1	3
Israel	22	9	10	12	42	48	22
Japan	0	0	0	0	0	0	0
Jordan	13	22	29	29	20	18	20
Kazakhstan	+..	+..	+..	0	0	0	0
Korea (Dem. People's Rep.)	…	…	0	…	…	…	…
Korea (Rep. of)	+..	19	3	14	18	10	4
Kuwait	0	0	0	0	0	0	0
Kyrgyzstan	…	67	+()	2	119	78	72
Laos	+..	+..	+..	+..	+..	+..	…
Lebanon	0	0	0	0	0	0	0
Malaysia	0	0	0	0	0	0	0
Maldives	…	…	…	0	0	0	…
Mongolia	18	…	23	34	65	154	72
Myanmar	+	2	9	1	6	9	7
Nepal	…	11	42	1	23	7	12
Oman	7	4	12	28	11	49	37
Pakistan	…	…	+()	+()	+()	+()	+()
Palestinian Auton. Territories	0	0	0	0	0	1	0
Philippines	+	+	+	+	629	546	350
Qatar	0	0	0	0	+..	0	0
Saudi Arabia	9	2	+..	+..	+..	+..	+..
Singapore	0	0	0	0	0	0	0
Sri Lanka	110	8	+	65	115	87	88
Syria	16	+..	+..	0	2	4	7
Tajikistan	32	10	99	112	59	56	70
Thailand	250	120	260	215	280	185	107
Turkmenistan	…	…	…	…	…	+..	…
United Arab Emirates	0	0	0	0	0	0	0
Uzbekistan	98	+..	+..	+..	…	…	…
Vietnam	5	1	23	6	2	+()	+()
Yemen	9	354	886	189	20	413	216

[a] Number of new outbreaks reported to OIE

0 Disease absent; +.. disease present but without quantitative data; + disease present with quantitative data but with an unknown number of outbreaks; … no information available; +() disease limited to one or more zones; ? disease suspected but not confirmed

Table 3.3 Incidence of rabies in animals in African countries (2005–2011) (OIE 2013)

	New outbreaks[a]						
Country	2005	2006	2007	2008	2009	2010	2011
Algeria	887	808	995	1,088	718	563	686
Angola	4	7	28	17	12	+	10
Benin	…	…	2	0	0	5	1
Botswana	32	25	48	57	39	29	29
Burkina Faso	5	2	+..	+..	+..	+..	+..
Burundi	+	…	…	+	+	3	…
Cameroon	5	1	4	1	?	4	1
Cape Verde	…	…	…	0	0	…	…
Central African Republic	+..	+..	+..	+..	16	10	+..
Chad	+..	+	…	…	…	4	14
Comoros	…	…	…	0	0	0	0
Congo (Dem. Rep. of the)	+..	+..	+	+..	+..	+..	5
Congo (Rep. of the)	…	…	…	…	…	…	…
Cote D'Ivoire	+..	+..	6	1	13	10	13
Djibouti	0	0	0	0	0	0	0
Egypt	0	0	0	0	0	0	0
Equatorial Guinea	…	…	…	…	?	?	?
Eritrea	1	1	1	1	5	0	…
Ethiopia	64	61	58	30	38	83	34
Gabon	…	12	10	12	10	1	3
Gambia	…	…	…	?	1	…	…
Ghana	13	23	10	31	21	31	26
Guinea	38	37	23	57	38	55	44
Guinea-Bissau	+..	?	?	?	?	?	?
Kenya	49	72	48	55	77	59	77
Lesotho	41	24	43	23	17	3	11
Libya	0	0	0	1	+..	+..	…
Madagascar	23	4	1.	+..	+..	7	9
Malawi	32	4	25	6	16	30	21
Mali	+..	+..	?	1	0	0	0
Mauritania	13	7	4	+..	14	11	11
Mauritius	0	0	0	0	0	0	0
Morocco	47	326	350	307	284	254	248
Mozambique	13	6	10	14	5	7	2
Namibia	216	154	72	32	90	175	207
Niger	…	0	0	+..	1	5	+()
Nigeria	3	1	2	23	24	5	11
Reunion (France)	0	0	0	0	0	0	0
Rwanda	…	14	22	12	3	33	32
Sao Tome and Principe	…	…	…	0	0	…	…
Senegal	1	1	1	0	1	2	18
Seychelles	…	…	…	…	…	0	0
Sierra Leone	…	…	…	…	0	+	+..

(continued)

Table 3.3 (continued)

Country	New outbreaks[a] 2005	2006	2007	2008	2009	2010	2011
Somalia	…	…	…	0	0	0	5
South Africa	290	472	392	488	522	401	295
Sudan	3	0	4	1	4	5	1
Swaziland	13	41	48	59	47	36	32
Tanzania	82	…	87	28	14	16	10
Togo	58	25	37	39	28	18	14
Tunisia	83	+	+	+	80	116	91
Uganda	11	?	?	?	+..	1	3
Zambia	…	33	50	106	125	96	+
Zimbabwe	234	…	121	61	38	128	184

[a] Number of new outbreaks reported to OIE
0 Disease absent; +.. disease present but without quantitative data; + disease present with quantitative data but with an unknown number of outbreaks; … no information available; +() disease limited to one or more zones; ? disease suspected but not confirmed

while raccoon dogs (*Nyctereutes procyonoides*) play a significant role in the epidemiology of rabies in the Baltic countries (Cliquet et al. 2010). In addition, distinct epidemiological cycles occur in certain bat species involving different lyssaviruses. Classical rabies has been eliminated in many European countries through implementation of oral rabies vaccination programmes. The majority of the Western European countries are now free of classical rabies, with reported rabies restricted to relatively rarer bat cases (European bat lyssaviruses type 1 and type 2). However, rabies is still prevalent in wildlife in several eastern member states of the European Union and adjacent non-member states.

Based on the data provided by the European countries to the Rabies Information System of the WHO Collaboration Centre for Rabies Surveillance and Research, the numbers of rabies cases in domestic animals, wildlife, bats, and human beings in Europe are shown in Table 3.4. The numbers of animals tested negative during the same period are shown in Table 3.5.

3.5 Rabies in North America

Rabies was most likely present in the New World before European colonisation. Reports of Spanish conquistadors dying after being bitten by vampire bats exist as early as 1514 (Baer 2007). However, canine rabies was most likely introduced after colonisation. Rabies epizootics associated with dogs were not reported until the early eighteenth century, but later on dogs remained the primary source of rabies in the USA until the mid-twentieth century. Subsequently, with the control of canine rabies, the epidemiology of rabies in the USA shifted to primary circulation and maintenance in wildlife species (Blanton et al. 2011).

Over the last 100 years, the situation of rabies in the USA has changed dramatically. The number of rabies-related human deaths in the USA has declined from more than 100 annually at the turn of the century to one or two per year in the 1990s, largely due to the availability and success of modern prophylaxis measures. Every year, it is estimated that 40,000 persons receive PEP against potential exposure to rabies (CDC 2012b).

Since 1995, 49 human rabies cases have been recorded in the USA (CDC 2012a). These are summarised in Table 3.6. Human fatalities associated with rabies occur mainly in the people who fail to seek medical assistance, usually because they were unaware of their exposure (Blanton et al. 2011).

Before 1960, the majority of animal rabies cases reported annually to CDC were in domestic

Table 3.4 Rabies cases in European countries (2001–2011) (Rabies Bulletin Europe 2012)

Country	Domestic animals	Wildlife excluding bats	Bat	Human cases	Total
Albania	8	9	0	0	17
Austria	4	24	0	0	28
Belarus	2,604	6,706	0	1	9,311
Belgium	1	0	0	0	1
Bosnia–Herzegovina	104	415	0	0	519
Bulgaria	58	224	0	0	282
Croatia	516	6,240	0	0	6,756
Cyprus	0	0	0	0	0
Czech Republic	2	36	1	0	39
Denmark	1	0	23	0	24
Estonia	328	1,780	0	0	2,108
Finland	1	0	1	0	2
France	11	0	51	0	62
Germany	9	172	107	6	294
Greece	0	0	0	0	0
Hungary	168	634	4	0	806
Iceland	0	0	0	0	0
Ireland	0	0	0	0	0
Italy	15	272	0	1	288
Latvia	649	3,026	0	1	3,676
Lithuania	1,747	6,021	0	0	7,768
Luxembourg	0	0	0	0	0
Macedonia	0	6	0	0	6
Malta	0	0	0	0	0
Moldova	323	179	0	0	502
Montenegro	29	173	0	0	202
Norway	0	0	0	0	0
Poland	758	4,489	61	0	5,308
Portugal	0	0	0	0	0
Romania	1,111	3,287	1	1	4,400
Russian Federation	15,143	12,754	5	84	27,986
Serbia	115	688	0	0	803
Slovak Republic	82	555	0	0	637
Slovenia	14	255	0	0	269
Spain	28	0	8	0	36
Sweden	0	0	0	0	0
Switzerland + Lichtenstein	1	0	1	0	2
The Netherlands	0	0	90	0	90
Turkey	2,013	234	0	0	2,247
Ukraine	11,269	8,614	11	9	19,903
UK	1	0	9	5	15
Total	37,113	56,793	373	108	94,387
%	39.3	60.2	0.4	0.1	100

animals, but now more than 90 % of these occur in wildlife. The principal rabies hosts today are wild carnivores and bats. Outbreaks of rabies infections in terrestrial mammals like raccoons, skunks, foxes, and coyotes are found in broad geographical regions across the USA (CDC 2012b).

Most people are exposed to rabies due to close contact with domestic animals, such as

Table 3.5 Animals tested negative in rabies surveillance in European countries (2001–2011) (Rabies Bulletin Europe 2012)

Country	Domestic animals	Wildlife excluding bats	Bat	Total
Albania	30	162	148	340
Austria	791	37,714	574	39,079
Belarus	171	40	0	211
Belgium	2,280	1,073	173	3,526
Bosnia–Herzegovina	152	70	0	222
Bulgaria	405	1,527	1	1,933
Croatia	5,318	23,239	81	28,638
Cyprus	0	0	0	0
Czech Republic	2,929	37,767	89	40,785
Denmark	22	13	100	135
Estonia	780	1,076	5	1,861
Finland	207	3,242	46	3,495
France	8,191	1,183	1,262	10,636
Greece	82	4	5	91
Hungary	4,385	39,670	59	44,114
Italy	4,262	25,795	237	30,294
Kosovo	22	18	0	40
Latvia	1,249	2,609	0	3,858
Lithuania	2,768	5,838	6	8,612
Luxembourg	24	137	0	161
Macedonia	2	164	0	166
Moldova	270	89	19	378
Montenegro	1	219	0	220
Poland	11,160	155,652	580	167,392
Portugal	0	0	0	0
Romania	112	102	0	214
Russian Federation	0	0	0	0
Serbia	1,256	846	5	2,107
Slovak Republic	2,547	20,612	26	23,185
Slovenia	835	10,252	611	11,698
Spain	102	72	69	243
Sweden	0	0	0	0
Switzerland + Lichtenstein	188	252	121	561
The Netherlands	62	48	825	935
Turkey	2,093	133	3	2,229
Ukraine	9,083	44,655	35	53,773
UK	179	75	5,599	5,853
Total	61,958	414,348	10,679	486,985
%	12.7	85.1	2.2	100

cats or dogs. While dogs have historically been associated with rabies transmission to humans, cats are more likely to be reported rabid in the USA. Cats are often in close contact with both humans and wild animals, implying that rabies may be more easily transmitted to humans from cats (CDC 2012b).

Rabies surveillance data of the USA and Puerto Rico for the period 2005–2010 has been presented in Table 3.7. In 2010, 48 states and Puerto Rico reported 6,153 cases of rabies in animals and 2 in humans (Blanton et al. 2011; CDC 2012b). Wild animals accounted for 92 % of reported cases of rabies in 2010. Raccoons were the most frequently

Table 3.6 Cases of rabies in human beings in the USA (1995–2011) (CDC 2012a)

Sr. No.	Date of death	Exposure history[a]	Rabies virus variant[c]
1	March 15, 1995	Unknown[b]	Bat, Msp
2	September 21, 1995	Unknown[b]	Bat, Tb
3	October 3, 1995	Unknown[b]	Bat, Ln/Ps
4	November 9, 1995	Unknown[b]	Bat, Ln/Ps
5	February 8, 1996	Dog bite – Mexico	Dog, Mexico
6	August 20, 1996	Dog bite – Nepal	Dog, SE Asia
7	October 15, 1996	Unknown	Bat, Ln/Ps
8	December 19, 1996	Unknown	Bat, Ln/Ps
9	January 5, 1997	Unknown[b]	Bat, Ln/Ps
10	January 18, 1997	Unknown[b]	Bat, Ef
11	October 17, 1997	Unknown[b]	Bat, Ln/Ps
12	October 23, 1997	Unknown[b]	Bat, Ln/Ps
13	December 31, 1998	Unknown	Bat, Ln/Ps
14	September 20, 2000	Unknown[b]	Bat, Tb
15	October 9, 2000	Dog bite – Ghana	Dog, Africa
16	October 10, 2000	Unknown[b]	Bat, Tb
17	October 25, 2000	Bat bite – MN	Bat, Ln/Ps
18	November 1, 2000	Unknown[b]	Bat, Ln/Ps
19	February 4, 2001	Unknown[b] – Philippines	Dog, Philippines
20	March 31, 2002	Unknown[b]	Bat, Tb
21	August 31, 2002	Unknown[b]	Bat, Ln/Ps
22	September 28, 2002	Unknown[b]	Bat, Ln/Ps
23	March 10, 2003	Unknown[b]	Raccoon, eastern USA
24	June 5, 2003	Bite	Dog/mongoose, Puerto Rico
25	September 14, 2003	Bite	Bat, Ln/Ps
26	February 15, 2004	Bite	Dog, Haiti
27	May 3, 2004	Bite (organ donor)	Bat, Tb
28	June 7, 2004	Liver transplant recipient	Bat, Tb
29	June 9, 2004	Kidney transplant recipient	Bat, Tb
30	June 10, 2004	Arterial transplant recipient	Bat, Tb
31	June 21, 2004	Kidney transplant recipient	Bat, Tb
32	Survived, 2004	Unknown[b]	Bat, unknown
33	October 26, 2004	Unknown[b]	Dog, El Salvador
34	September 27, 2005	Unknown[b]	Bat, unknown
35	May 12, 2006	Unknown[b]	Bat, Tb
36	November 2, 2006	Bite	Bat, Ln/Ps
37	December 14, 2006	Bite	Dog, Philippines
38	October 20, 2007	Bite	Bat, unknown
39	March 18, 2008	Bite – Mexico	Fox, Tb-related
40	November 30, 2008	Bite	Bat, Ln/Ps
41	Survived, 2009	Unknown[b]	Bat, unknown
42	October 20, 2009	Unknown[b]	Bat, Ps
43	November 11, 2009	Unknown[b]	Bat, Ln/Ps
44	November 20, 2009	Bite	Dog, India
45	August 21, 2010	Bite	Bat, Mexico, Ds
46	January 10, 2011	Unknown	Bat, Ps

(continued)

Table 3.6 (continued)

Sr. No.	Date of death	Exposure history[a]	Rabies virus variant[c]
47	Survived, 2011	Unknown	Unknown
48	July 20, 2011	Bite	Dog, Haiti
49	August 31, 2011	Bite	Dog, Afghanistan

[a]Data for exposure history are reported only when the biting animal was available and tested positive for rabies or when plausible information was reported directly by the patient (if lucid or credible) or when a reliable account of an incident consistent with rabies exposure (e.g. dog bite) was reported by an independent witness (usually a family member)
[b]In some instances where the exposure history is unknown, there may have been known or inferred interaction which, especially for bats, could have involved an unrecognised bite
[c]Variants of the rabies virus associated with terrestrial animals in the USA are identified with the name of the reservoir animal (dog or dog/coyote in all cases shown) followed by the name of the most definitive geographical entity (usually the country) from which the variant has been identified. Variants of the rabies virus associated with bats are identified with the name(s) of the species of bat(s) in which they have been found to be circulating. Because information regarding the location of the exposure and the identity of the exposing animal are almost always retrospective, and much information is frequently unavailable, the location of the exposure and the identity of the animal responsible for the infection are often limited to deduction
Ln/Ps = *Lasionycteris noctivagans* or *Pipistrellus subflavus*, the silver-haired bat or the eastern pipistrelle; Msp = *Myotis*, species unknown; Tb = *Tadarida brasiliensis*, the Brazilian (Mexican) free-tailed bat; Ef = *Eptesicus fuscus*, the big brown bat; Ds = *Desmodus rotundus*, the vampire bat

Table 3.7 Rabies surveillance data in the USA and Puerto Rico (2005–2010) (Blanton et al. 2006, 2007, 2008, 2009, 2010, 2011)

Type of rabid species	2005	2006	2007	2008	2009	2010
Cases of rabies in animals	6,417	6,940	7,258	6,841	6,694	6,153
Human cases	1	3	1	2	4	2
Total wild animals cases	5,923	6,393	6,776	6,369	6,185	5,666
Raccoons	2,534	2,615	2,659	2,389	2,327	2,246
Skunks	1,478	1,494	1,478	1,589	1,603	1,448
Foxes	376	427	489	454	504	429
Bats	1,408	1,692	1,973	1,806	1,625	1,430
Domestic animals	494	547	482	471	505	487
Rabid cats	269	318	274	294	300	303
Rabid dogs	76	79	93	75	81	69
Rabid cattle	93	82	57	59	74	71

reported rabid wildlife species in the year 2010 (2,246 raccoons, 36.5 % of all rabid animals during 2010), followed by 1,448 skunks (23.5 %), 1,430 bats (23.2 %), 429 foxes (6.9 %), 303 cats (4.9 %), 71 cattle (1.1 %), and 69 dogs (1.1 %). Other wild animals included rodents and lagomorphs (1.8 %) (Blanton et al. 2011). Domestic species accounted for about 8 % of all rabid animals reported in the USA in 2010. Approximately 1.1 % of cats and 0.3 % of dogs tested for rabies were found positive (CDC 2012b).

In Canada too, rabies represents a serious threat although human cases are rarely reported. One case of human rabies was recorded in the country during 1993–2002 (Belotto et al. 2005). Thereafter, one human fatality due to rabies was recorded each in the year 2003 and 2007 (Krebs et al. 2004; Blanton et al. 2008). The status of human and animal rabies in Canada during 2005–2010 is summarised in Table 3.8. During 2010, no human cases of rabies were reported; however, there were 123 laboratory-confirmed cases of rabies involving animals (Blanton et al. 2011). Ninety-three per cent (n = 114) of the cases involved rabid wildlife, 1.6 % (2) involved rabid livestock, and 5.7 % (7) involved rabid cats

Table 3.8 Cases of rabies in Canada (2005–2010) (Blanton et al. 2006, 2007, 2008, 2009, 2010, 2011)

Type of rabid species	2005	2006	2007	2008	2009	2010
Domestic and wild animals	248	229	273	235	145	123
Human cases	0	0	1	0	0	0
Wild animals	214	176	243	204	122	114
Livestock	18	34	19	16	11	2
Companion animals	16	19	11	15	12	7
Bats	94	72	93	61	55	48
Raccoons	3	5	59	27	0	0
Skunks	94	84	78	99	49	60
Foxes	18	14	13	15	13	6
Dogs	12	13	7	12	9	3
Cats	4	6	3	3	3	4
Bovines	16	26	15	12	8	1
Equines	2	7	2	0	0	1

and dogs. No rabid wolves were reported in Canada in 2010, compared with 5 in 2009. Rabid foxes (6), bats (48), dogs (3), and cattle (1) were reported in the year 2010. The corresponding numbers of these animals during the year 2009 were 13, 55, 9, and 8, respectively. The reported number of rabid skunks was 60, cats 4, and equids 1 in 2010, while the corresponding figures of these during 2009 were 49, 3, and 0, respectively (Blanton et al. 2011).

3.6 Rabies in Latin America

In Latin America, two distinct epidemiological cycles of rabies circulating in dogs and bats have been recognised since early colonial times. Dog rabies is suspected to have been present in Mexico since 1709 (Malaga-Alba 1957) while records in South America date to the early nineteenth century (Steele 1975). Leans (2011) analysed the epidemiological trends of human and canine rabies cases during 1970–2009 in Latin America. He observed that the number of human cases was very high, at times even greater than 300 per year, up to 1990s which gradually declined to 19 in the year 2009. According to the information available at the Epidemiological Information System, 56 human rabies cases were reported in the year 2011 while the average for the past one decade was 56 human cases (PAHO 2012). The corresponding number of canine rabies cases in the year 2011 stood at 466 while the average for the previous decade was 989.

There has been substantial reduction in human and canine rabies cases due to systematic control programmes but rabies continues to pose a real challenge in the region. During the period 2000–2009, total 462 cases of human rabies were recorded (PAHO Rabies Information System 2011; Leans 2011). These were transmitted by different animal species including dogs (239), vampire bats (149), non-hematophagous bats (11), nonspecified bats (15), cats (9), cattle and horses (4), wild carnivores (10), and unspecified sources (25). The incidence of rabies in animals reported to the OIE by different countries in the Americas (excluding USA and Canada) during the years 2005–2011 has been summarised in Table 3.9.

3.7 Rabies in Australia and Oceania

Australia is currently free from classical rabies. Only two imported human cases have been reported between 1900 and 1995 in travellers who returned from endemic areas, one in 1987 and another in 1990 (CDC 1988; Department of Health, Australia 2012). Subsequently, two human cases of Australian bat lyssavirus infection were

Table 3.9 Incidence of rabies in animals in Latin American countries (2005–2011) (OIE 2013)

	New outbreaks[a]						
Country	2005	2006	2007	2008	2009	2010	2011
Argentina	2	27	39	22	7	24	58
Aruba	…	…	…	…	…	0	0
Barbados	0	…	0	…	…	0	0
Belize	11	2	2	3	0	5	0
Bolivia	231	23	30	330	75	43	35
Brazil	1,496	1,388	1,096	1,135	1,135	913	938
Cayman Islands	0	0	…	…	…	…	…
Chile	…	0	1	0	0	30	42
Colombia	103	111	92	119	152	156	100
Costa Rica	4	2	1	0	3	1	3
Cuba	21	47	32	81	74	42	34
Dominica	…	…	…	0	…	…	…
Dominican Republic	27	80	16	89	103	78	95
Ecuador	12	4	11	32	26	27	53
El Salvador	174	241	97	55	4	18	4
French Guiana	0	0	0	0	1	0	0
Grenada	…	?	…	?	+..	+..	…
Guadeloupe (France)	0	0	0	0	0	0	0
Guatemala	35	28	77	102	142	95	96
Guyana	+()	+()	+()	+()	+()	+()	+()
Haiti	+..	+..	+..	+..	+..	+..	+..
Honduras	0	+()	0	1	18	3	…
Jamaica	0	0	0	0	0	0	…
Martinique (France)	0	0	0	0	0	0	0
Mexico	249	47	268	205	335	321	214
Nicaragua	1	4	1	0	1	0	0
Panama	4	29	8	25	7	8	17
Paraguay	+..	+	+..	+..	21	46	62
Peru	55	104	93	106	81	104	92
St. Kitts and Nevis	0	…	…	…	…	…	…
St. Vincent and the Grenadines	…	0	0	0	0	0	…
Suriname	0	0	0	0	0	0	0
Trinidad and Tobago	1	1	1	0	0	3	2
Uruguay	0	0	26	30	30	12	0
Venezuela	27	12	34	54	32	26	11

[a]Number of new outbreaks reported to OIE
0 Disease absent; +.. disease present but without quantitative data; + disease present with quantitative data but with an unknown number of outbreaks; … no information available; +() disease limited to one or more zones; ? disease suspected but not confirmed

reported, one from Northern New South Wales (1996) and the other from Rockhampton in Queensland (1998). These persons had a history of bites and scratches from a bat and both developed fatal encephalitis and died (Department of Health, Australia 2012). Rabies of bat origin is thus an emerging infectious disease in the region and the risk of human exposure rises with the increasing human contact with Australian bat environments.

Table 3.10 Incidence of rabies in animals in Oceania (2005–2011) (OIE 2013)

	New outbreaks[a]						
Country	2005	2006	2007	2008	2009	2010	2011
Australia	0	0	0	0	0	0	0
Fiji	…	…	0	0	0	0	0
French Polynesia	0	0	0	0	0	0	0
Kiribati	…	…	…	0	…	…	…
Micronesia (Federated States)	…	…	…	0	0	0	0
New Caledonia	0	0	0	0	0	0	0
New Zealand	0	0	0	0	0	0	0
Papua New Guinea	…	…	…	0	0	0	0
Samoa	0	…	…	0	0	0	…
Tonga	…	…	…	…	…	…	…
Tuvalu	…	0	0	0	…	…	…
Vanuatu	0	0	0	0	0	0	0
Wallis and Futuna Islands	…	…	0	…	…	…	…

[a]Number of new outbreaks reported to OIE
0 Disease absent; … no information available

As revealed from the data reported to the OIE concerning rabies in animals, the disease is generally absent in Oceania region (OIE 2013), but in some cases, the information on the disease is yet not available (Table 3.10).

3.8 Bat Rabies

The significance of bats as sources of rabies infection has been increasingly appreciated, and new information has been accumulating rapidly during recent years. Rabies in flying mammals (Chiroptera) is known to be widespread; however, it is neither transmitted by the same species nor caused by the same virus in all parts of the world (FLI 2012). Bats are the principal reservoirs for most of the recognised lyssavirus species (Table 2.1) and are suspected as hosts of other putative species (Kuzmin et al. 2010, 2011). Rabies virus, which circulates in bats and other mammals, is known to circulate in bats only in the Americas, whereas globally, it circulates in carnivores. In the Old World, bats maintain circulation of other lyssavirus species, such as Lagos bat virus, Duvenhage virus, European bat lyssaviruses type 1 and type 2, Australian bat lyssavirus, Aravan virus, Khujand virus, Irkut virus, West Caucasian bat virus, and Shimoni bat virus. For these viruses, bats are the principal hosts, with only a few spillover infections documented in other mammals (Kuzmin et al. 2011). It is not known which lyssaviruses circulate in bats of northern Africa and southern Asia because surveillance data from developing countries is very limited. However, historical reports along with more recent serological findings indicate that bats do maintain lyssavirus circulation in these territories (Kuzmin et al. 2011).

3.8.1 Bat Rabies in the Americas

Bats are the source of most human rabies deaths in the USA and Canada. As seen from Table 3.6, during the period 1995–2011, out of 49 human cases of rabies in the USA, 35 were associated with bats. Out of total 24,298 bat specimens examined during the year 2010, 1,430 (5.9 %)

Table 3.11 Species of bats tested rabies positive in the USA during 2010 (Blanton et al. 2011)

Bat species (common name)
Antrozous pallidus (desert pallid bat)
Eptesicus fuscus (big brown bat)
Lasionycteris noctivagans (silver-haired bat)
Lasiurus borealis (red bat)
Lasiurus cinereus (hoary bat)
Lasiurus ega (southern yellow bat)
Lasiurus intermedius (northern yellow bat)
Lasiurus seminolus (seminole bat)
Lasiurus xanthinus (western yellow bat)
Myotis austroriparius (southeastern myotis)
Myotis evotis (long-eared myotis)
Myotis lucifugus (little brown bat)
Myotis spp. (not further speciated)
Myotis thysanodes (fringed myotis)
Myotis volans (long-legged myotis)
Myotis yumanensis (Yuma myotis)
Nycticeius humeralis (evening bat)
Nyctinomops macrotis (big free-tailed bat)
Parastrellus hesperus (canyon bat)
Perimyotis subflavus (tricoloured bat)
Tadarida brasiliensis (Mexican free-tailed bat)
Unspeciated

were positive for rabies (Blanton et al. 2011). The number of rabies-positive bat specimens was even more during the previous years 2006 (1,692), 2007 (1,973), 2008 (1,806), and 2009 (1,625) (Blanton et al. 2006, 2007, 2008, 2009, 2010, 2011). The corresponding numbers of rabies-positive bats reported in Canada were 72, 93, 61, 55, and 48 in the years 2006, 2007, 2008, 2009, and 2010, respectively (Krebs et al. 2004, 2005; Blanton et al. 2006, 2007, 2008, 2009, 2010, 2011). The species of bats that tested positive for rabies in the USA in 2010 as reported by Blanton et al. (2011) are listed in Table 3.11. Out of total 1,430 rabies-positive bat specimens, 648 were unspeciated.

The analysis of 1,147 human rabies cases encountered in the Americas (including North America and Latin America) during 1993–2002 has revealed that the transmitting animal species included hematophagous bats (62 cases), non-hematophagous bats (27 cases), and unidentified species of bats (79 cases) (Belotto et al. 2005). Another report covering the period 2000–2009 reveals even greater public health threat posed by the bats in Latin America. During this period, out of 462 cases of human rabies, vampire bats were implicated in 149 cases, non-hematophagous bats in 11 cases, and nonspecified bat species in 15 cases (PAHO Rabies Information System 2011; Leans 2011). Apart from it, the economic losses due to vampire bat rabies in livestock are tremendous (Kuzmin et al. 2011).

In a similar study in Brazil, among the 863 cases of rabies diagnosed in bats between 2001 and 2007, 424 (49.1 %) were non-hematophagous bats, 250 (29 %) were hematophagous bats, and 189 (21.9 %) were of unidentified species (PAHO 2008; Sodre et al. 2010). Sodre et al. (2010) analysed the database (1996–2009) and developed an updated list of bat species positive for rabies in Brazil. The new list of rabies-positive bats consists of 41 species, belonging to 25 genera and three families: Phyllostomidae (43.9 %), Vespertilionidae (29.3 %), and Molossidae (26.8 %). These have been presented in Table 3.12.

3.8.2 Bat Rabies in Europe

In Europe, though the risk of possible exposure to bat lyssaviruses is low, sporadic human rabies cases following a bat bite have been described. The first confirmed case of European bat lyssaviruses type 1 associated with a bat bite in Europe was reported in Ukraine in 1977 and another fatal infection in Russia in 1985. A fatal case of European bat lyssaviruses type 2 infection in a Swiss biologist who had multiple bat bites was recorded in Finland in 1985. The second confirmed case of this infection following exposure to bats occurred in Scotland in 2002 (Rabies Bulletin Europe 2012).

From 1977–2010, total 959 cases of bat rabies were detected in Europe and reported to the WHO Collaborating Centre for Rabies Surveillance and Research in Germany. The majority (more than 90 %) of positive bats originated from Denmark, followed by the

Table 3.12 List of Brazilian bat species positive for rabies (1996–2009) (Sodre et al. 2010)

Phyllostomidae	Vespertilionidae	Molossidae
Anoura caudifer	*Eptesicus brasiliensis*	*Eumops auripendulus*
Anoura geoffroyi	*Eptesicus diminutus*	*Eumops glaucinus*
Artibeus fimbriatus	*Eptesicus furinalis*	*Eumops perotis*
Artibeus lituratus	*Histiotus velatus*	*Cynomops abrasus*
Artibeus planirostris	*Lasiurus blossevillii*	*Cynomops planirostris*
Carollia perspicillata	*Lasiurus cinereus*	*Molossops neglectus*
Chrotopterus auritus	*Lasiurus ega*	*Molossus molossus*
Desmodus rotundus	*Lasiurus egregius*	*Molossus rufus*
Diaemus youngi	*Myotis albescens*	*Nyctinomops laticaudatus*
Diphylla ecaudata	*Myotis levis*	*Nyctinomops macrotis*
Glossophaga soricina	*Myotis nigricans*	*Tadarida brasiliensis*
Lonchorhina aurita	*Myotis riparius*	
Lophostoma brasiliense		
Micronycteris megalotis		
Phyllostomus hastatus		
Platyrrhinus lineatus		
Trachops cirrhosus		
Uroderma bilobatum		

Netherlands, Germany, and Poland. Bat rabies was also reported from France, Spain, Switzerland, Great Britain, the Czech Republic, Slovakia, Hungary, Ukraine, and Russia. European bat lyssaviruses type 1 has a specific association with the Serotine bat (*Eptesicus serotinus*, in Spain *E. isabellinus*), while type 2 is associated with the species of Myotis bats (*M. daubentonii* and *M. dasycneme*) and has been isolated from bats in the Netherlands, UK, Switzerland, Germany, and Finland. West Caucasian bat lyssavirus was isolated from a common bent-winged bat (*Miniopterus schreibersi*) and Bokeloh bat lyssavirus from a Natterer's bat (*Myotis nattereri*) recently from Germany (Rabies Bulletin Europe 2012).

Transmission of bat rabies to terrestrial mammals (spillover), though a rare incident, represents a potential risk. In 1998 and 2002, European bat lyssaviruses type 1-induced rabies was detected in sheep in Denmark. The first spillover to wildlife species was confirmed in 2001 in Germany. France also reported the infections in two cats in 2003 and 2007, respectively (Rabies Bulletin Europe 2012).

3.8.3 Bat Rabies in Australia

In Australia, both the larger flying foxes (fruit bats) and the smaller insectivorous (micro) bats have been found to carry Australian bat lyssavirus. The virus was identified in 1996 in a sick black flying fox (*Pteropus alecto*). The second case was diagnosed retrospectively in another bat of the same species, sampled in 1995 with signs of unusual aggressiveness (Fraser et al. 1996; Kuzmin et al. 2011). Later the infection was documented in each of the four flying fox species, present in continental Australia. Furthermore, a genetically divergent variant of the virus was discovered in insectivorous bats *Saccolaimus flaviventris* (Gould et al. 2002; Kuzmin et al. 2011). Studies suggest that this lyssavirus is widely distributed in Australia, and it is therefore assumed that all Australian bats have the potential to carry and transmit the virus. There is no evidence that lyssaviruses in bats can establish and spread among terrestrial animals, although isolated cases in humans may occur on rare occasions. Two such cases have been reported in Australia (Department of Health, Australia 2012).

3.8.4 Bat Rabies in Africa

A variety of bat lyssaviruses have been documented in Africa. Lagos bat virus, first documented in Nigeria in 1956 (Boulger and Porterfield 1958), was further isolated in many sub-Saharan countries (Kuzmin et al. 2008a, 2010). Moreover, in 1999, it was imported into France with fruit bats *Rousettus aegyptiacus* captured in Togo or Egypt (Aubert 1999). Fruit bats of several species serve as reservoir hosts for this virus, with infrequent spillover infections documented in dogs, cats, and a mongoose (Markotter et al. 2006). Another divergent lyssavirus, Shimoni bat virus, was isolated from insectivorous bat *Hipposideros commersoni* in Kenya in 2009. This virus demonstrates similarity to Mokola virus and Lagos bat virus, but cannot be included into any of these species (Kuzmin et al. 2010). Recently, serological reactivity to West Caucasian bat lyssavirus was detected in *Miniopterus* bats of several species from Kenya (Kuzmin et al. 2008b).

3.8.5 Bat Rabies in Asia

Data on rabies in Asian bats are limited because of lack of a suitable surveillance system. Only a few investigators reported presumable rabies virus isolates of bat origin in Asia till recently, but these were not corroborated (Kuzmin et al. 2006). However, in the last 10 years, evidence of lyssavirus maintenance in Southeast Asian Chiropterans has emerged from surveillance in Cambodia, Thailand, Bangladesh, and the Philippines (Kuzmin et al. 2006; Robertson et al. 2011). Neutralising antibodies associated with lyssaviruses have been detected in sera from both regional mega- and microbats, suggesting that Asian bats maintain lyssaviruses like their counterparts in Europe, Africa, Australia, and the Americas (Robertson et al. 2011).

At least two bat-associated human rabies or rabies-like cases have been reported during the past decade in Northeast China. It prompted a study of the prevalence of lyssaviruses in bats in the region which led to the recovery of an Irkut virus isolate with high pathogenicity in experimental mice from the brain of a northeastern bat, *Murina leucogaster* (Liu et al. 2013). This is likely to boost the interest in the role of bats in lyssavirus transmission in the continent.

References

Aubert MFA (1999) Rabies in individual countries, France. Rabies Bull Europe 23(2):6

Baer GM (2007) The history of rabies. In: Jackson AC, Wunner WH (eds) Rabies, 2nd edn. Academic, London, pp 1–22

Belotto A, Leanes LF, Schneider MC, Tamayo H, Correa E (2005) Overview of rabies in Americas. Virus Res 111:5–12

Blanton JD, Krebs JW, Hanlon CA, Rupprecht CE (2006) Rabies surveillance in the United States during 2005. J Am Vet Med Assoc 229:1897–1911

Blanton JD, Hanlon CA, Rupprecht CE (2007) Rabies surveillance in the United States during 2006. J Am Vet Med Assoc 231:540–556

Blanton JD, Palmer D, Robertson K, Rupprecht CE (2008) Rabies surveillance in the United States during 2007. J Am Vet Med Assoc 233:884–897

Blanton JD, Robertson K, Palmer D, Rupprecht CE (2009) Rabies surveillance in the United States during 2008. J Am Vet Med Assoc 235:676–689

Blanton JD, Palmer D, Rupprecht CE (2010) Rabies surveillance in the United States during 2009. J Am Vet Med Assoc 237:646–657

Blanton JD, Palmer D, Dyer J, Rupprecht CE (2011) Rabies surveillance in the United States during 2010. J Am Vet Med Assoc 239:773–783

Boulger LR, Porterfield JS (1958) Isolation of a virus from Nigerian fruit bats. Trans R Soc Trop Med Hyg 52:421–424

CDC (1988) Imported human rabies- Australia, 1987. Morb Mortal Wkly Rep 37(22):351–353

CDC (2012a) Rabies. Centers for Disease Control and Prevention. http://www.cdc.gov/rabies/. Accessed 30 Mar 2012

CDC (2012b) The burden of rabies. Centers for Disease Control and Prevention. http://www.cdc.gov/Features/dsRabies/. Accessed 8 Apr 2012

Cleaveland S, Fevre EM, Kaare M, Coleman PG (2002) Estimating human rabies mortality in the United Republic of Tanzania from dog bite injuries. Bull WHO 80:304–310

Cliquet F, Freuling C, Smreczak M, Van der Poel WHM, Horton D, Fooks AR, Robardet E, Picard-Meyer E, Müller T (2010) Development of harmonised schemes for monitoring and reporting of rabies in animals in the European Union. Scientific Report submitted to European Food Safety Authority (EFSA). http://www.efsa.europa.eu/en/supporting/doc/67e.pdf. Accessed 10 Mar 2012

Davis PL, Rambaut A, Bourhy H, Holmes EC (2007) The evolutionary dynamics of canid and mongoose rabies virus in Southern Africa. Arch Virol 152:1251–1258

Department of Health, Australia (2012) Rabies and Australian bat lyssavirus infection. Department of Health, Victoria, Australia. http://ideas.health.vic.gov.au/bluebook/rabies.asp. Accessed 13 Apr 2012

Deray RA (2009) Country report: Philippines. In: Hanh NTH (ed) Proceedings of the second international conference of Rabies in Asia Foundation (RIACON 2009), Hanoi, 9–11 Sept 2009

FLI (2012) Bats – Species protection and rabies in Europe – Information leaflet. Federal Research Institute for Animal Health, WHO Collaborating Centre for Rabies Surveillance and Research, Friedrich-Loeffler-Institute, Wusterhausen, Germany. http://www.who-rabies-bulletin.org/about_rabies/Bats/Information_Bat%20rabies_%20Europe.pdf. Accessed 30 Mar 2012

Fraser GC, Hooper PT, Lunt RA, Gould AR, Gleeson LJ, Hayatt AD, Russell GM, Kattenbelt JA (1996) Encephalitis caused by a lyssavirus in fruit bats in Australia. Emerg Infect Dis 2:327–331

Gongal G, Wright AE (2011) Human rabies in the WHO Southeast Asia Region: forward steps for elimination. Adv Prev Med. doi:10.4061/2011/383870

Gould AR, Kattenbelt JA, Gumley SG, Lunt RA (2002) Characterisation of an Australian bat lyssavirus variant isolated from an insectivorous bat. Virus Res 89:1–28

Harischandra PAL (2009a) Country report of rabies control in Sri Lanka 2008. In: Hanh NTH (ed) Proceedings of the second international conference of Rabies in Asia Foundation (RIACON 2009), Hanoi, 9–11 Sept 2009

Harischandra PAL (2009b) Dog rabies control in Sri Lanka. In: Hanh NTH (ed) Proceedings of the second international conference of Rabies in Asia Foundation (RIACON 2009), Hanoi, 9–11 Sept 2009

Health Protection Agency (2012) Rabies risks in terrestrial animals, by country. Health Protection Agency. http://www.hpa.org.uk/Topics/InfectiousDiseases/InfectionsAZ/Rabies/Guidelines/rabrabiescountryrisks/. Last reviewed 17 May 2011. Accessed 23 Apr 2012

Health Protection Scotland (2012) Rabies country risk table (last updated 12 March 2012). Health Protection Scotland. http://www.documents.hps.scot.nhs.uk/giz/rabies/rabies-table-2012-03.pdf. Accessed 23 Apr 2012

Hien NT (2009) Rabies situation in Vietnam, 2008. In: Hanh NTH (ed) Proceedings of the second international conference of Rabies in Asia Foundation (RIACON 2009), Hanoi, 9–11 Sept 2009

Inoue S (2009) Rabies prevention in Japan. In: Hanh NTH (ed) Proceedings of the second international conference of Rabies in Asia Foundation (RIACON 2009), Hanoi, 9–11 Sept 2009

Joshi DD (2009) Rabies outbreaks review: Recorded cases and National Strategic Control Plan in Nepal. In: Hanh NTH (ed) Proceedings of the second international conference of Rabies in Asia Foundation (RIACON 2009), Hanoi, 9–11 Sept 2009

Knobel DL, Cleaveland S, Coleman PG, Fevre EM, Meltzer MI, Miranda ME, Shaw A, Zinsstag J, Meslin FX (2005) Re-evaluating the burden of rabies in Africa and Asia. Bull WHO 83:360–368

Krebs JW, Mandel EJ, Swerdlow DL, Rupprecht CE (2004) Rabies surveillance in the United States during 2003. J Am Vet Med Assoc 225:1837–1849

Krebs JW, Mandel EJ, Swerdlow DL, Rupprecht CE (2005) Rabies surveillance in the United States during 2004. J Am Vet Med Assoc 227:1912–1925

Kuzmin IV, Neizgoda M, Carroll DS, Keeler N, Hossain MJ, Breiman RF, Ksiazek TG, Rupprecht CE (2006) Lyssavirus surveillance in bats, Bangladesh. Emerg Infect Dis 12:486–488

Kuzmin IV, Niezgoda M, Franka R, Agwanda B, Markotter W, Beagley JC, Urazova OY, Breiman RF, Rupprecht CE (2008a) Lagos bat virus in Kenya. J Clin Microbiol 46:1451–1461

Kuzmin IV, Niezgoda M, Franka R, Agwanda B, Markotter W, Beagley JC, Urazova OY, Breiman RF, Rupprecht CE (2008b) Possible emergence of West Caucasian bat virus in Africa. Emerg Infect Dis 14:1887–1889

Kuzmin IV, Mayer AE, Niezgoda M, Markotter W, Agwanda B, Breiman RF, Rupprecht CE (2010) Shimoni bat virus, a new representative of the Lyssavirus genus. Virus Res 149:197–210

Kuzmin IV, Bozick B, Guagliardo SA, Kunkel R, Shak JR, Tong S, Rupprecht CE (2011) Bats, emerging infectious diseases, and the rabies paradigm revisited. Emerg Health Threats J 4:7159. doi:10.3402/ehtj.v4i0.7159

Leans LF (2011) New approaches to rabies elimination in Latin America. Presentation: rabies elimination in the 21st century? Public Health Grand Rounds. http://www.cdc.gov/about/grand-rounds/archives/2011/pdfs/PHGRRabies20Jan201010am.pdf. Accessed 30 Aug 2012

Liu Y, Zhang S, Zhao J, Zhang F, Hu R (2013) Isolation of Irkut virus from a *Murina leucogaster* bat in China. PLoS Negl Trop Dis 7(3):e2097. doi:10.1371/journal.pntd.0002097

Malaga-Alba A (1957) Rabies in wildlife in Middle America. J Am Vet Med Assoc 130:386–390

Mallewa M, Fooks AR, Banda D, Chikungwa P, Mankhambo L, Molyneux E, Molyneux ME, Solomon T (2007) Rabies encephalitis in malaria-endemic area, Malawi, Africa. Emerg Infect Dis 13:136–139

Markotter W, Kuzmin I, Rupprecht CE, Randles J, Sabeta CT, Wandeler AI, Nel LH (2006) Isolation of Lagos bat virus from water mongoose. Emerg Infect Dis 12:1913–1918

Nel LH, Thomson GR, Von Teichman BF (1993) Molecular epidemiology of rabies virus in South Africa. Onderstepoort J Vet Res 60:301–306

OIE (2013) World Animal Health Information Database (WAHID) Interface. World Organisation for Animal Health. http://web.oie.int/wahis/public.php?page=home. Accessed 25 May 2013

PAHO (2008) Epidemiological Information System. Pan-American Health Organization/World Health Organization. http://siepi.panaftosa.org.br/anuais.aspx. Cited from Sodre et al. (2010)

PAHO (2012) Epidemiological Information System (SIEPI), Pan American Health Organization, Panaftosa – PAHO/WHO. http://siepi.panaftosa.org.br/Panel.aspx?Idioma=i. Accessed 12 Apr 2012

Panichabhongse P (2009) Rabies in Thailand. In: Hanh NTH (ed) Proceedings of the second international conference of Rabies in Asia Foundation (RIACON 2009), Hanoi, 9–11 Sept 2009

Rabies Bulletin Europe (2012) Rabies Information System of the WHO Collaboration Centre for Rabies Surveillance and Research. http://www.who-rabies-bulletin.org. Accessed 25 May 2013

PAHO Rabies Information System (2011) SIRVERA. www.panaftosa.org.br. Updated December 2010. Cited from Leans (2011)

Rahman S (2009) Rabies in Bangladesh. In: Hanh NTH (ed) Proceedings of the second international conference of Rabies in Asia Foundation (RIACON 2009), Hanoi, 9–11 Sept 2009

Rinzin K (2009) Control of animal rabies in Bhutan. In: Hanh NTH (ed) Proceedings of the second international conference of Rabies in Asia Foundation (RIACON 2009), Hanoi, 9–11 Sept 2009

Robertson K, Lumlertdacha B, Franka R, Petersen B, Bhengsri S, Henchaichon S, Peruski LF, Baggett HC, Maloney SA, Rupprecht CE (2011) Rabies-related knowledge and practices among persons at risk of bat exposures in Thailand. PLoS Negl Trop Dis 5(6):e1054. doi:10.1371/journal.pntd.0001054

Salahuddin N (2009) Rabies in Pakistan. In: Hanh NTH (ed) Proceedings of the second international conference of Rabies in Asia Foundation (RIACON 2009), Hanoi, 9–11 Sept 2009

Sodre MM, da Gama AR, de Almeida MF (2010) Updated list of bat species positive for rabies in Brazil. Rev Inst Med Trop São Paulo 52(2):75–81. http://dx.doi.org/10.1590/S0036-46652010000200003. Accessed 18 Jan 2012

Steele JH (1975) History of rabies. In: Baer GM (ed) The natural history of rabies, vol I. Academic, New York, pp 1–29

Sudarshan MK, Madhusudana SN, Mahendra BJ, Rao NS, Ashwath Narayana DH, Abdul Rahman S, Meslin FX, Lobo D, Ravikumar K, Gangaboraiah (2007) Assessing the burden of human rabies in India: results of a national multi-center epidemiological survey. Int J Infect Dis 11:29–35

Swanepoel R, Barnard BJ, Meredith CD, Bishop GC, Bruckner GK, Foggin CM, Hübschle OJ (1993) Rabies in southern Africa. Onderstepoort J Vet Res 60:325–346

Talbi C, Holmes EC, de Benedictis P, Faye O, Nakouné E, Gamatié D, Diarra A, Elmamy BO, Sow A, Adjogoua EV, Sangare O, Dundon WG, Capua I, Sall AA, Bourhy H (2009) Evolutionary history and dynamics of dog rabies virus in western and central Africa. J Gen Virol 90:783–791

Tang Q (2009) Rabies in China. In: Hanh NTH (ed) Proceedings of the second international conference of Rabies in Asia Foundation (RIACON 2009), Hanoi, 9–11 Sept 2009

Undraa B (2009) Rabies in Mongolia. In: Hanh NTH (ed) Proceedings of the second international conference of Rabies in Asia Foundation (RIACON 2009), Hanoi, 9–11 Sept 2009

von Teichman BF, Thomson GR, Meredith CD, Nel LH (1995) Molecular epidemiology of rabies virus in South Africa: evidence for two distinct virus groups. J Gen Virol 76:73–82

Vong S (2009) Assessing the burden of rabies in Cambodia: challenges and opportunities. In: Hanh NTH (ed) Proceedings of the second international conference of Rabies in Asia Foundation (RIACON 2009), Hanoi, 9–11 Sept 2009

WHO (2012) Rabies. World Health Organization. www.who.int. Accessed 10 Mar 2012

WHO Global Vaccine Research Forum (2006) Epidemiology of rabies in Asia. http://www.who.int/vaccine_research/about/gvrf/Miranda_presentation.pdf. Accessed 15 Aug 2012

4 Rabies Manifestations and Diagnosis

Abstract

All mammals are susceptible to rabies but there are variations in the disease manifestations among various animal species and even within the species. The animals may exhibit furious form of the disease or dumb/paralytic form. In general, rabies virus causes acute encephalitis with fatal outcome. The incubation period of rabies is quite variable in different cases as it is influenced by several factors. In humans, it is generally 1–3 months but may vary from less than one week to over a year. Because of the wide variation and non-characteristic signs, reliable diagnosis of rabies is based on identifying the virus or some of its specific components. Fluorescent antibody test (FAT) is the most widely used method for diagnosing rabies in animals and humans. Intra vitam diagnosis of rabies may require several tests; no single test is sufficient. Samples of saliva, serum, spinal fluid, and skin biopsies of hair follicles at the nape of the neck may be used for laboratory diagnosis. Serological tests are useful mainly to evaluate the immunogenicity of human and animal rabies vaccines.

4.1 Manifestations in Animals

All mammals are susceptible to rabies. These include pet animals, livestock, wild animals, and bats. Different species show different signs of the disease. There are variations in the manifestation of disease even within the same species. All the signs of rabies may not always be exhibited by all the animals. Moreover, some of the signs may be so subtle that they can go unnoticed. In general, rabies virus causes acute encephalitis in all warm-blooded hosts and the outcome is almost always fatal. One of the first signs of rabies in an animal is a change in behaviour. It is usually reflected by a normally calm animal turning aggressive or a usually active animal looking depressed or dull. In case of wild animals, a rabid animal can lose fear of humans, and nocturnal animals might be seen during daylight hours.

The severity and the site of the lesions largely decide the clinical picture of the disease. Depending on these, the disease may exhibit signs of irritative (furious form) or paralytic (dumb or paralytic form) phenomena. Many cases lie somewhere between these two extreme forms of the clinical picture of rabies (Radostits et al. 2007). The source of the virus may also cause variations in the major manifestations, mania or paralysis. Virus from vampire bats almost always causes the paralytic form. 'Fixed'

S.R. Garg, *Rabies in Man and Animals*, DOI 10.1007/978-81-322-1605-6_4,

virus that has been modified by serial intracerebral passage causes ascending paralysis in contrast to 'street' virus, which more commonly causes the furious form. The site of infection and size of inoculum may also influence the clinical course. There is also geographical difference in the proportion of animals affected by the furious or paralytic form of the disease. In the Americas most cases are paralytic. In Africa and India, most cases in farm animals display the furious form (Radostits et al. 2007).

4.1.1 Incubation Period

The incubation period of rabies is quite variable in different cases. It is influenced by the amount of virus transmitted, virus strain, site of inoculation, host immunity, and the severity of bite. The incubation period is shorter in case the site of bite is near to the head and where the site has more nerves in comparison to the cases where the rabid animal inflicts a bite on the extremities. Similarly, deep and multiple wounds infected with higher concentration of rabies virus may result in a more severe and rapid onset of disease. In dogs and cats, the incubation period may be around 10 days to 6 months; most cases become apparent between 2 weeks and 3 months (CFSPH 2009). In most species, the incubation period in naturally occurring cases is about 3 weeks but varies from 2 weeks to several months, although incubation periods of 5–6 months have been observed in cattle and dogs. Experimentally, the average incubation period has been reported as 15 days in cattle, 10 days in sheep, and 12 days in horses. Unvaccinated animals have been reported to have shorter incubation and clinical duration of disease than the vaccinated animals (Hudson et al. 1996a, b; Radostits et al. 2007).

4.1.2 Clinical Signs in Dogs

The first symptoms of rabies in the dogs may be nonspecific. This stage is called as prodromal phase and the signs include restlessness, anorexia or an increased appetite, vomiting, a slight fever, dilation of the pupils, hyperreactivity to stimuli, and excessive salivation. There may be change in the behaviour and temperament of the animal. The affected animal may become either more aggressive or dull, opposite to its normal behaviour. The pet may turn unresponsive to the pet owner and may prefer sitting in isolation. On the other hand, it may turn unusually affectionate, contrary to its normal response. Noticing a sudden change of behaviour may help in suspecting the disease in early stages.

The prodromal signs usually last for 2–5 days and then may lead to further progression of the disease (CFSPH 2009). The disease may appear in two forms: furious form and dumb form.

4.1.2.1 Furious Form of Rabies

Furious form of rabies is very common in dogs and the animal becomes quite excited and restless. A rabid dog becomes dangerously aggressive and bites objects like its own chain, stones, paper, wood, and metal and even may show signs of snapping at imaginary objects. There may be unusual bark and aimless wandering. Later, there is drooling of saliva due to paralysis of muscles of deglutition. Partial paralysis of vocal cords leads to change in tone of bark to howl. The dog may not recognise its owner. In the terminal stage, there is muscular incoordination and paralysis of limbs and trunk. Death occurs mostly due to respiratory paralysis and convulsions.

4.1.2.2 Dumb Form of Rabies

Dumb form is the paralytic form of rabies which is characterised by progressive paralysis. In some cases it may develop without any noticeable signs of the furious form of the disease. Throat and masseter muscles become paralysed and the animal may be unable to swallow. This causes saliva to accumulate with possible drooling and foaming (Fig. 4.1). There may be facial paralysis or the lower jaw may drop. Dumb form of rabies is less common in dogs. The phase of excitement is short or absent in the dumb form. The dog has a dull or vacant expression and prefers to sit isolated in a corner (Fig. 4.2). It may respond to its owner's call but there is tendency of forgetfulness (Fig. 4.3). Paralysis begins with the muscles of

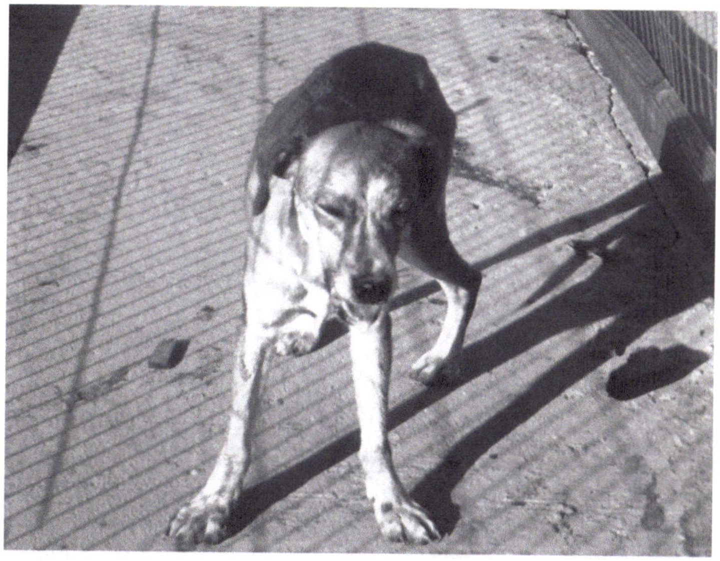

Fig. 4.1 A rabid dog with saliva dripping from the mouth (Photo courtesy: CDC)

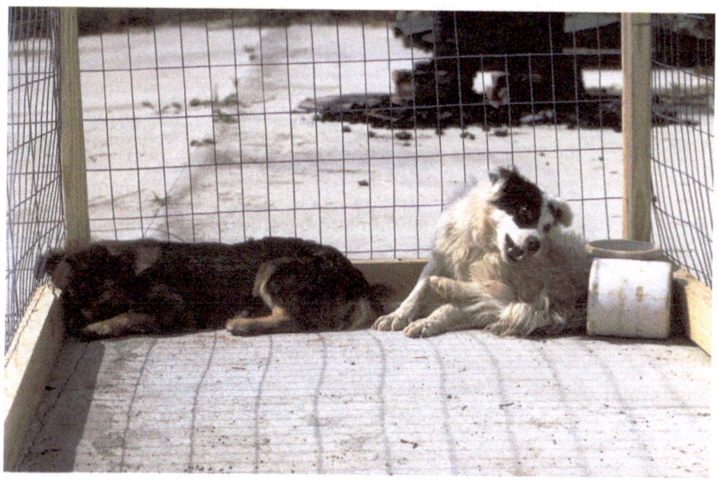

Fig. 4.2 Two dogs afflicted with dumb rabies, manifested as depression, and self-imposed isolation (Photo courtesy: CDC)

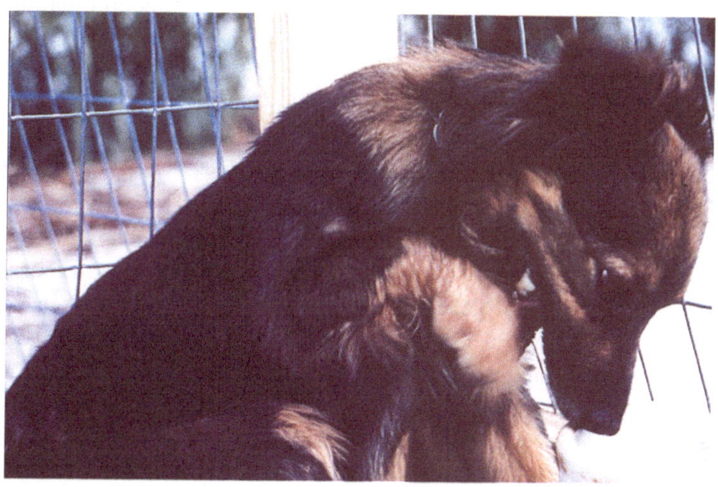

Fig. 4.3 A dog afflicted with dumb rabies, manifested as depression, lethargy, and a seemingly overly tame disposition (Photo courtesy: CDC)

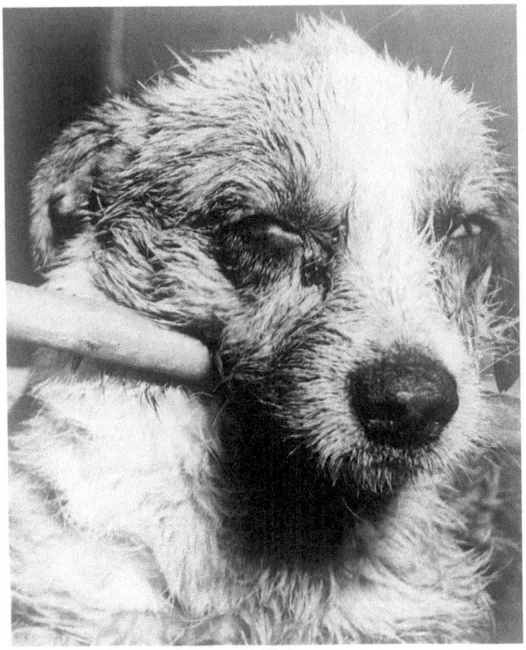

Fig. 4.4 Close-up of a dog's face during late-stage 'dumb' paralytic rabies (Photo courtesy: CDC, Barbara Andrews)

head and neck region (Fig. 4.4). The animal has difficulty in swallowing. This is often mistaken as bone stuck in the mouth and the owner out of ignorance tries to help the dog and gets exposed to infection. General paralysis results in death of the animal usually in 3–5 days.

4.1.3 Clinical Signs in Cats

In a cat, the disease is usually of furious type. The cat may strike at the air with its forepaws as if it were catching mice. Paralysis of the hind part begins 2–4 days after the symptoms of excitement, and the animal generally dies in 3–5 days due to convulsions and respiratory paralysis.

4.1.4 Clinical Signs in Livestock

In domestic animals, rabies should be suspected if there is a sudden change in disposition and failure to eat or drink or if the animal becomes paralysed or runs into objects (Shultz 2004). Ruminants may separate from the herd and stop ruminating. Subsequently, there is ataxia, incoordination, and ascending spinal paresis or paralysis. The clinical picture of rabies in different species of the farm animals has been vividly described by Radostits et al. (2007).

4.1.5 Clinical Signs in Cattle

Rabies in cattle may be manifested either in furious form or in paralytic form. Cattle may appear unusually alert. Convulsions can occur, particularly in the terminal stages. In the final stages, there is incoordination and ascending paralysis. The animal usually dies 4–8 days after the onset of the clinical signs (CFSPH 2009).

In an experimental study, major clinical findings of the disease included excessive salivation (100 %); behavioural change (100 %); muzzle tremors (80 %); vocalisation (bellowing 70 %); aggression, hyperesthesia, and/or hyperexcitability (70 %); and pharyngeal paralysis (60 %). The furious form occurred in 70 % cases. Average course of the disease has been recorded as 3.7 days (Hudson et al. 1996b; Radostits et al. 2007).

4.1.5.1 Furious Form of Rabies

In furious form of rabies, the animal has a tense, alert appearance. It is hypersensitive to sounds and movement. In some cases, it violently attacks other animals or inanimate objects, but these attacks are often badly directed and reveal incoordination of gait. The animal shows loud bellowing and produces a characteristically hoarse sound. Sexual excitement is also common, bulls often attempting to mount inanimate objects (Radostits et al. 2007). There is very wide variation in the clinical signs; hence, any animal known to be exposed to rabies or showing nervous signs should be considered rabid until proved otherwise. Severe clinical signs may be evident for 24–48 h, and the animal then collapses suddenly in a paralysed state, dying usually within a few hours. Body temperatures are usually normal but may be elevated to 39.5–40.5 °C (103–105 °F) in the early stages by muscular activity. There is variation in appetite too.

Some animals do not eat or drink, although they may take food into the mouth. The inability to swallow is apparent. Other animals may eat normally until the terminal stages. The course of the disease may vary from 1 to 6 days (Radostits et al. 2007).

4.1.5.2 Paralytic Form of Rabies

Early signs in the paralytic form of the disease include knuckling of the hind fetlocks, sagging, and swaying of the hindquarters while walking and often deviation or flaccidity of the tail to one side. Decreased sensation, most evident over the hindquarters, is one of the best diagnostic criteria in the detection of rabies. Tenesmus, with paralysis of the anus, resulting in the sucking in and blowing out of air, is a characteristic finding but it may be transient or absent (Radostits et al. 2007). It usually occurs late in the incoordination stages just before the animal becomes recumbent. Drooling of saliva is one of the most constant findings. There are yawning movements which are more accurately described as voiceless attempts to bellow. When paralysis occurs, the animal becomes recumbent and unable to rise. Bulls in this stage often have paralysis of the penis. Death usually occurs 48 h after the recumbency develops and after a total course of 6–7 days.

4.1.6 Clinical Signs in Sheep and Goats

Clinical picture of rabies in sheep is similar to that in cattle. Rabies may occur in a number of animals at one time due to the ease with which a number of sheep can be bitten by a dog or fox (Radostits et al. 2007). Major clinical findings in an experimental study included muzzle and head tremors (80 %), aggressiveness, hyperexcitability and hyperesthesia (80 %), trismus (60 %), salivation (60 %), vocalisation (60 %), and recumbency (40 %). The furious form occurred in 80 % of sheep. The average course of the disease in experimental study was 3.25 days (Hudson et al. 1996b).

Sudden falling after violent exertion, muscle tremor, and salivation are characteristic signs. Some animals show sexual excitement, attacking humans or each other, and vigorous wool pulling. Excessive bleating does not occur. Most sheep are quiet and anorectic. In one large outbreak of rabies in sheep, deaths occurred between 17 and 111 days after exposure. Goats are commonly aggressive, and continuous bleating is common (Radostits et al. 2007).

4.1.7 Clinical Signs in Horses

In naturally occurring cases in horses, the initial clinical findings may include abnormal postures, frequent whinnying, aggressiveness and kicking, biting, colic, sudden onset of lameness in one limb followed by recumbency the next day, high-stepping gait, ataxia, apparent blindness, and violent head tossing. Lameness or weakness in one leg may be the first sign observed, but the usual pattern of development starts with lassitude, then passes to sternal recumbency and lateral recumbency, followed by paddling convulsions and terminal paralysis (Radostits et al. 2007). Most recorded cases in horses lack distinctive nervous signs initially but incline to the paralytic form of the disease. In an experimental study, the average duration of disease has been determined as 5.5 days, and muzzle tremors were the most frequently observed and most common initial signs (Hudson et al. 1996a; Radostits et al. 2007). Other clinical findings included pharyngeal paresis (71 %), ataxia or paresis (71 %), and lethargy or somnolence (71 %). The furious form occurred in 43 % of cases, some of which began as the dumb form. The paralytic form was not observed.

In a series of 21 confirmed cases in horses studied by Green et al. (1992), the clinical findings at the time of initial examination included ataxia and paresis of the hindquarters (43 %), lameness (24 %), recumbency (14 %), pharyngeal paralysis (10 %), and colic (10 %). The major clinical findings observed over the course of hospitalisation included recumbency (100 %), hyperesthesia (81 %), loss of tail and anal sphincter tone (57 %), 38.5 °C fever (52 %), and ataxia and paresis of the hindquarters (52 %). Mean survival time after the onset of clinical signs was 4.47 days (range, 1–7 days). Clinical findings of the furious form of rabies, such as aggressiveness (biting), compulsive circling, and abnormal vocalisation, were evident in only two horses. In furious form, the animals become excited and vicious and they bite and kick (Radostits et al. 2007).

4.1.8 Clinical Signs in Pigs

The clinical findings in pigs are extremely variable and only one or two of the classical findings may occur. Pigs manifest excitement and a tendency to attack or dullness and incoordination. Affected sows show twitching of the nose, rapid chewing movements, excessive salivation, and clonic convulsions. They may walk backwards. There is paralysis in terminal stage and death occurs 12–48 h after the onset of signs (Radostits et al. 2007).

4.1.9 Signs of Rabies in Wild Animals

Change in behaviour of wild animals such as loss of fear of man or unusual friendliness should be viewed with suspicion of rabies. Nocturnal animals may show abnormal activity during daytime and may attack humans. In the furious form of rabies, there is unprovoked aggression and some animals may attack anything that moves or even inanimate objects. The affected animal may appear disoriented or uncoordinated, or wander aimlessly. It may stumble or fall. Paralysis often begins in the hind legs or throat. Paralysis of the throat muscles can cause the animal to bark, whine, drool, choke, or froth at the mouth. Vocalisations ranging from chattering to shrill scream are observed (Shultz 2004). Skunks, raccoons, and foxes usually display furious rabies. Bats often display dumb rabies. Unable to fly, they may be found on the ground (Shultz 2004). This can be very risky for children, who are more likely to handle wild animals than adults.

4.2 Manifestations in Humans

In humans, the incubation period is a few days to several years. Typically it is 1–3 months but may vary from less than 1 week to over a year. The length of the incubation period depends on factors such as the amount of virus inoculated, the degree of innervation at the site of viral entry, and the proximity of the bite to the central nervous system (CNS) (WHO 2010).

The disease in the beginning appears with nonspecific symptoms. This stage is characterised with headache, anxiety, restlessness, fever, and often pain or paraesthesia at the wound site. As the virus spreads through the CNS, progressive fatal encephalomyelitis develops and an encephalitic (furious) form or a paralytic (dumb) form may predominate (CFSPH 2009; WHO 2010). Neural symptoms of the disease include excessive salivation, excitation, agitation, aggression, and abnormal behaviour (Fig. 4.5). Violent spasm of the gullet, pharynx, and larynx causes difficulty in swallowing of water and other fluids which is characterised by hydrophobia or aerophobia or both. The patient also becomes highly sensitive to noise and fearful of light (photophobia). These symptoms usually progress towards paralysis, coma, and death. In the terminal stages, there is respiratory paralysis, cardiac arrest, and death.

Paralytic (dumb) form is characterised by generalised paralysis. Paralytic rabies, which may represent as many as 30 % of the total human cases, is characterised by generalised paralysis. This form of disease runs a less dramatic and usually longer course than the furious form but it is ultimately fatal too (CFSPH 2009; WHO 2010).

4.3 Diagnostic Procedures

Rapid and accurate diagnosis of rabies is very important in prevention and control of rabies. Because the signs of the disease, particularly in the early stages, are not characteristic and may vary greatly between species and even between animals of the same species, the clinical observations

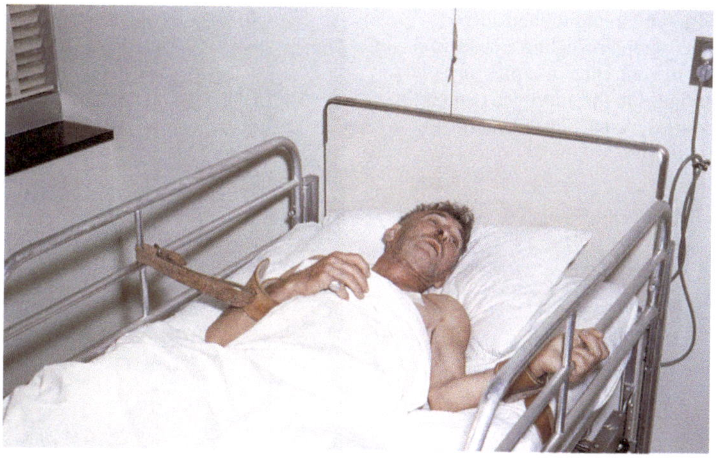

Fig. 4.5 A hospitalised human rabies victim in restraints (Photo courtesy: CDC)

may only lead to a suspicion of rabies but no confirmation. The only way to undertake a reliable diagnosis of rabies is to identify the virus or some of its specific components using laboratory tests (OIE Terrestrial Manual 2011). Laboratory tests help to determine whether or not an animal is rabid and to take decision accordingly regarding timely administration of the postexposure treatment. It also guides about the necessity of instituting epizootic control measures in an area. Rapid results may save a patient from unnecessary physical and psychological trauma and financial burdens, if the animal is not rabid (CDC 2012). Confirmation of positive rabies cases also provides epidemiological information of the disease and aids in development of rabies control programmes. Considering the nature of the disease, it is very essential that laboratory tests for rabies are adequately standardised, rapid, sensitive, specific, economical, and reliable (CDC 2012).

Several laboratory techniques are available that vary in their efficiency, specificity, and reliability. They are classically applied to brain tissue, but they can also be applied with variable sensitivity and specificity to other organs (e.g. salivary glands). As rabies virus is rapidly inactivated, refrigerated diagnostic specimens should be sent to the laboratory by the fastest means.

Diagnosis in Animals In animals, rabies is diagnosed using the direct fluorescent antibody test (FAT), which looks for the presence of rabies virus antigens in brain tissue. Diagnosis can be made after detection of rabies virus from any part of the affected brain, but in order to rule out rabies, the test must include tissue from at least two locations in the brain, preferably the brain stem and cerebellum (CDC 2012). The animal needs to be euthanised for the test. Collection of the brain sample from the suspected animal and its shipment to a diagnostic laboratory takes long time though the conduct of the test requires about 2 h only (CDC 2012).

Diagnosis in Humans During infection, the rabies virus is concealed from immune surveillance by its intraneuronal location, and antibody responses in serum and cerebrospinal fluid (CSF) are unpredictable and rarely detected before the disease has much progressed. Consequently, no tests are available to diagnose rabies infection in humans before the onset of clinical disease. The clinical diagnosis may be difficult unless the signs of hydrophobia or aerophobia are present (WHO 2010, 2012).

For intra vitam diagnosis of rabies at the stage of clinical manifestations in humans, several tests are necessary; no single test is sufficient. Tests are performed on samples of saliva, serum, spinal fluid, and skin biopsies of hair follicles at the nape of the neck. Saliva can be tested by virus isolation or reverse transcription followed by polymerase chain reaction (RT-PCR). Serum and spinal fluid are tested for antibodies to rabies virus. Skin biopsy specimens are examined for rabies antigen in the cutaneous nerves at the base of hair follicles (CDC 2012).

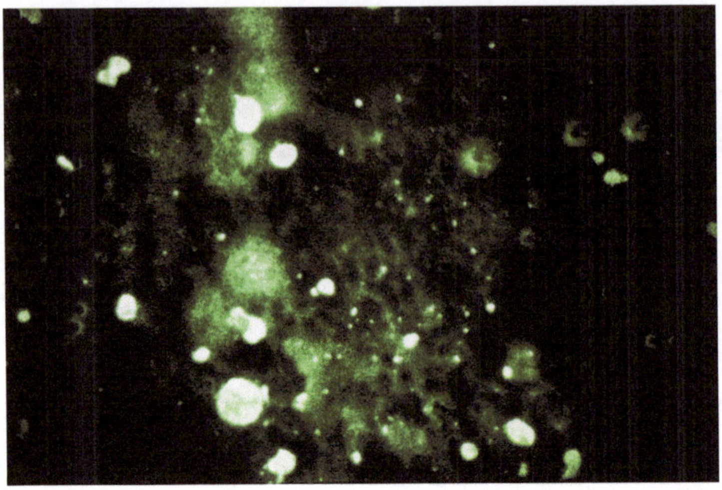

Fig. 4.6 Immunofluorescent micrograph revealing a positive result for the presence of rabies virus antigens in the specimen (Photo courtesy: CDC, Dr. Tierkel)

On post-mortem, the standard diagnostic technique is to detect rabies virus antigen in brain tissue by FAT (WHO 2012). A rapid tissue culture isolation test may also be used. A direct rapid immunohistochemical test is also available to detect rabies virus antigen in brain specimens.

Several new techniques and protocols have been proposed for rabies diagnosis; however, the reported number of laboratory-confirmed human rabies cases remains limited, particularly in Asia and Africa, resulting in underestimates of the real impact of the disease.

4.3.1 Identification of Rabies Virus or Its Specific Components

Identification of causative virus or some of its components in the specimen provides reliable diagnosis of rabies. The most widely used test for rabies diagnosis is FAT, which is recommended by both WHO and OIE, and is sensitive, specific, and cheap (OIE Terrestrial Manual 2011). In cases of inconclusive results from FAT, or in all cases of human exposure, further tests such as cell culture or mouse inoculation (MI) test on the same sample or repeat FAT on other samples are recommended. This is particularly important where sample autolysis is confirmed or suspected (OIE Terrestrial Manual 2011). Several other molecular techniques are also available that can be used as supplementary or confirmatory tests.

4.3.1.1 Fluorescent Antibody Test (FAT)

FAT is now the most widely used method for diagnosing rabies infection in animals and humans. The test is based on the observation that animals infected by rabies virus have rabies virus proteins (antigen) present in their tissues. Because rabies is present in nervous tissue (and not in blood as in many other viruses), the ideal tissue to test for rabies antigen is brain. The test is based on microscopic examination, under ultraviolet light, of impressions, smears, or frozen sections of brain or nervous tissue after treatment with antirabies serum or globulin conjugated with fluorescein isothiocyanate (FITC). Examination of impressions or smears of tissue samples from Ammon's horn and brain stem is recommended. Smears prepared from a composite sample of brain tissue are fixed in 100 % high-grade cold acetone for at least 20 min, air dried, and then stained with a drop of specific conjugate for 30 min at 37 °C. Commercially available antirabies fluorescent conjugates include polyclonal or monoclonal antibodies (MAb), specific to the entire virus or to the rabies nucleocapsid protein, conjugated to a fluorophore such as FITC. Labelled antibody upon incubation with rabies-suspect brain tissue binds to rabies antigen. Unbound antibody can be washed away and areas where antigen is present can be visualised as fluorescent-apple-green areas using a fluorescence microscope by trained personnel (Fig. 4.6). If rabies virus is absent, there will be no staining (OIE Terrestrial Manual 2011; WHO 2012; CDC 2012).

The test is accurate, and results can often be obtained within 30 min of receipt of the specimen, although for routine purposes a period of 2–4 h is desirable for the fixation in cold acetone (WHO 2012).

FAT is recommended by both WHO and OIE. This 'gold-standard' test may be used directly on a smear and can also be used to confirm the presence of rabies antigen in cell culture or in brain tissue of mice that have been inoculated for diagnosis. FAT gives reliable results on fresh specimens within a few hours in more than 95–99 % of cases. The test is sensitive, specific, and cheap (OIE Terrestrial Manual 2011).

The technique is highly sensitive in fresh specimens; however, it may also be performed on fixed specimens. The specimen should be treated with one or more proteolytic enzymes such as trypsin or pepsin before staining to unmask the antigenic sites. The sensitivity of the test using fixed specimens has been reported to be 90–100 % of that obtained using fresh specimens. It is recommended that fresh tissue be examined where possible. When specimens are received in 50 % glycerol-saline, it is imperative that the tissue be washed several times in saline before staining (WHO 2012).

4.3.1.2 Cell Culture Test

Samples containing small amounts of rabies virus may be difficult to confirm as rabies positive by routine methods. Virus replication in cell cultures such as mouse neuroblastoma cells and baby hamster kidney (BHK) cells increases the virus concentration without the use of animals. Cell culture tests may be undertaken in multi-well plastic plates, on multichambered glass slides, or on glass cover slips. After passage, the cells are examined by FAT. The cell culture technique is helpful in avoiding the use of laboratory animals and is less expensive and gives more rapid results in comparison to the MI test (OIE Terrestrial Manual 2011; CDC 2012; WHO 2012).

4.3.1.3 Mouse Inoculation (MI) Test

In this test, mice are inoculated intracerebrally with homogenate of brain material including brainstem (e.g. cortex, Ammon's horn, thalamus, medulla oblongata). The mice are observed daily for 28 days, and every dead mouse is examined for rabies using FAT. MI test may not be necessary and should be replaced with cell culture test wherever a validated and reliable cell culture unit exists in the laboratory. However, it is quite useful under the situations where skills and facilities for cell culture are not available (OIE Terrestrial Manual 2011).

4.3.1.4 Other Methods of Amplification of Virus Components

Apart from cell culture and MI techniques, several other molecular methods are available to amplify the small amounts of rabies virus in specimens which otherwise may be difficult to confirm by routine methods. RT-PCR, PCR-enzyme linked immunosorbent assay (PCR-ELISA), hybridisation in situ, and real-time PCR may help in rapid detection of viral RNA.

Another method for amplifying the nucleic acid portion of rabies virus uses biochemical techniques. With this procedure, rabies virus RNA can be enzymatically amplified as DNA copies. Rabies RNA can be copied into a DNA molecule using reverse transcriptase (RT). The DNA copy of rabies can then be amplified using PCR. This technique can confirm FAT results and can detect rabies virus in saliva and skin biopsy samples.

4.3.1.5 Histopathological Examination of Specimens

Prior to the availability of the current diagnostic methods, rabies diagnosis was made using histopathological examination of biopsy or autopsy tissues for the histopathological evidence of rabies encephalomyelitis. This method involves examining brain tissue and meninges by staining and microscopy. The signs of rabies encephalitis include mononuclear infiltration, perivascular cuffing of lymphocytes or polymorphonuclear cells, lymphocytic foci, Babes nodules consisting of glial cells, and Negri bodies (CDC 2012). Negri bodies correspond to the aggregation of viral proteins that are regarded as pathognomonic lesion, but the presence of Negri bodies is variable and their absence does not rule out the suspicion

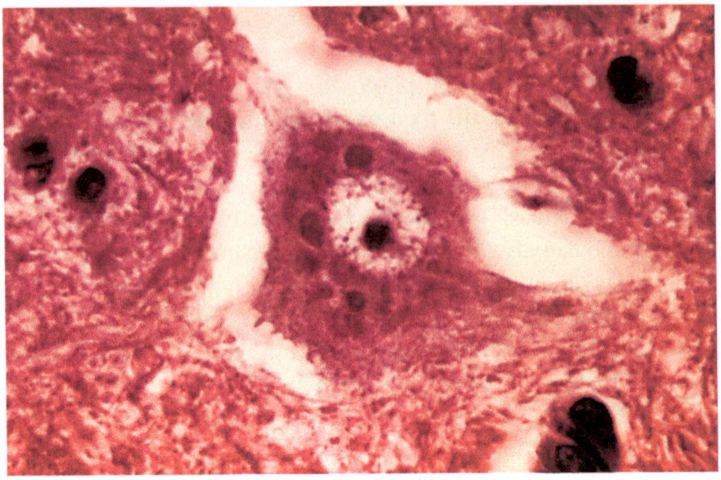

Fig. 4.7 Micrograph depicting Negri bodies and histopathological changes associated with rabies encephalitis. H&E stain (Photo courtesy: CDC, Dr. Daniel P. Perl)

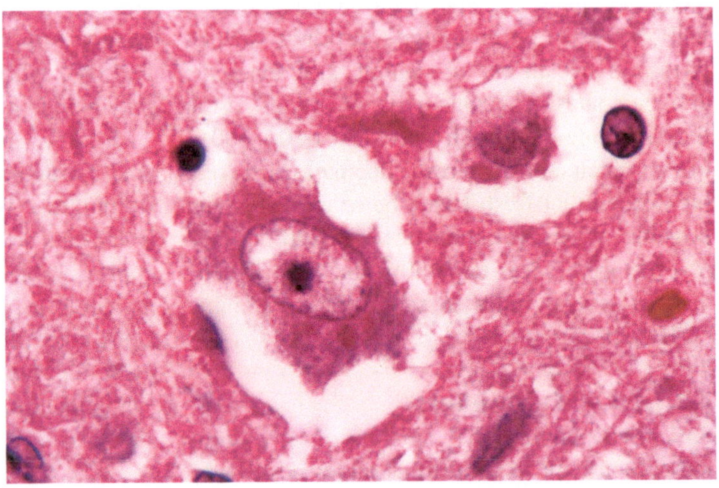

Fig. 4.8 Micrograph of brain tissue from a rabies encephalitis patient displaying Negri bodies within the neuronal cytoplasm. H&E stain (Photo courtesy: CDC, Dr. Daniel P. Perl)

of rabies (Figs. 4.7, 4.8, and 4.9). Thus, histopathological staining for Negri bodies is neither as sensitive nor as specific as other tests. Techniques that stain sections of paraffin-embedded brain tissues are time-consuming, less sensitive, and more expensive than FAT. These methods are no longer recommended for routine diagnosis (OIE Terrestrial Manual 2011; CDC 2012).

4.3.1.6 Immunohistochemistry (IHC)

Immunohistochemical tests constitute the only histological methods specific to rabies. These are more sensitive than histopathological staining methods, such as hematoxylin and eosin and Sellers stains. These provide sensitive and specific means to detect rabies in formalin-fixed tissues. Like FAT, these procedures use specific antibodies to detect rabies virus inclusions. The techniques use enzyme-labelling systems that increase sensitivity. In addition, MAb may be used to detect rabies virus variants (OIE Terrestrial Manual 2011; CDC 2012).

A rapid immunohistochemical test (RIT) to detect rabies virus antigen has been developed by incorporating various components of existing immunoperoxidase techniques (Niezgoda and Rupprecht 2006). Like the direct FAT, RIT is performed on brain touch impressions, but the product of the reaction can be observed by light microscopy, and rabies virus antigen appears as

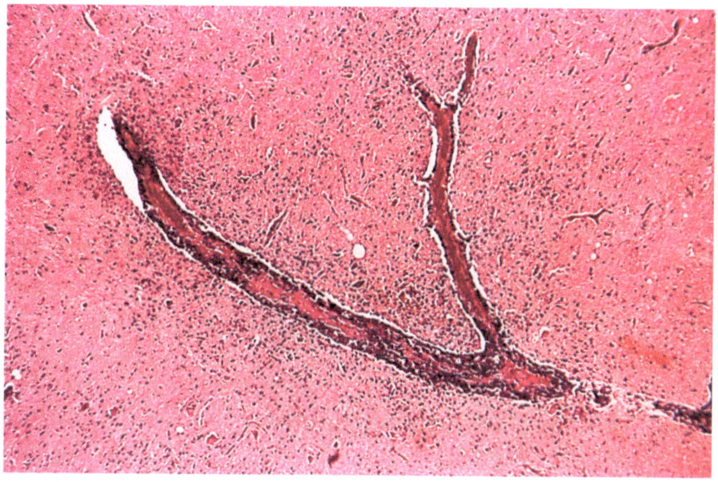

Fig. 4.9 Micrograph depicting perivascular cuffing due to the perivascular accumulation of inflammatory cell infiltrates. H&E stain (Photo courtesy: CDC, Dr. Daniel P. Perl)

magenta inclusions against a blue neuronal background. Modifications of a former indirect test have led to a direct test (dRIT) that uses a cocktail of highly concentrated and purified biotinylated antinucleocapsid MAb produced in vitro in a direct staining approach and allows a diagnosis to be made in <1 h.

The sensitivity and specificity of dRIT have been shown to be equivalent to those of the FAT. The test is simple, requires no specialised equipment or infrastructure, and can be successfully performed on samples preserved in glycerol solution for 15 months or frozen for 24 months and in variable conditions of preservation (Lembo et al. 2006). Although further laboratory and field evaluations are required, the test is quite promising and has great potential for use under field conditions and in the countries with limited diagnostic resources.

4.3.1.7 Rapid Rabies Enzyme Immunodiagnosis (RREID)

RREID has been developed based on ELISA used for the detection of rabies virus nucleocapsid antigen in brain tissue. In this test, microplates are coated with purified IgG and an IgG–peroxidase conjugate is used to react with immunocaptured antigen. However, the test has been found to be less sensitive in comparison to FAT; hence it should not replace FAT in the laboratories where FAT is already performed (WHO 2012). RREID is a simple and relatively cheap technique, which can be especially useful for epidemiological surveys. It may be used to examine partially decomposed tissue specimens for evidence of rabies infection, but it cannot be used with specimens that have been fixed in formalin. Since the antigen can be visualised with the naked eye, the test can be carried out in laboratories that do not have the necessary equipment for FAT (WHO 2012).

4.3.1.8 Electron Microscopy

The ultra structure of viruses can be examined by electron microscopy. Using this method, the structural components of viruses and their inclusions can be observed in detail. Rabies virus is in the family of rhabdoviruses which are seen as bullet-shaped particles when viewed with an electron microscope (Fig. 2.1).

4.3.1.9 Virus Identification Techniques

Typing of the virus can provide useful epidemiological information. The use of MAb helps in identifying various lyssavirus serotypes. Virus identification is useful in determining the geographical origin of strains, distinguishing between field and vaccine strains, and differentiating rabies viruses isolated from terrestrial animal species from those isolated from bat species. Although MAb are mainly used for epidemiological investigations, they have been found to be very useful for rabies diagnosis in certain circumstances, such as imported cases of human rabies and rabies associated with uncertain exposure, and also routinely in countries where large-scale programmes for oral vaccination of foxes are underway to establish that no infections are caused by the vaccine strain. Other techniques of virus typing involve the use of nucleic acid probes or PCR, followed by DNA sequencing of genomic areas (OIE Terrestrial Manual 2011; WHO 2012).

4.3.2 Serological Tests for Rabies Antibodies

Serological tests are useful mainly to evaluate the immunogenicity of human and animal rabies vaccines. In accordance with the WHO recommendations, 0.5 IU per ml of rabies antibodies is the minimum measurable antibody titre considered to represent a level of immunity in humans that correlates with the ability to protect against rabies infection. The same measure is used in dogs and cats to confirm a satisfactory response to vaccination. In case of animals, the test is useful in determining responses to vaccination, either in domestic animals prior to international travel or in wildlife populations following oral immunisation. Serological surveys have also been used to provide information on dynamics of lyssaviruses in bats although standardisation of serological tests for bats is still needed (OIE Terrestrial Manual 2011).

Serum neutralisation assays are used to determine the potency of rabies serum and immunoglobulin for postexposure treatment and to evaluate the immunogenicity of human and, to a lesser degree, animal rabies vaccines.

4.3.2.1 Mouse Neutralisation Test

Mouse neutralisation test (MNT) and the plaque reduction assay were recommended as the standard procedures at the seventh meeting of the WHO Expert Committee on Rabies, but plaque reduction methods have now been superseded by fluorescent focus inhibition tests, which are more convenient. Virus neutralisation test in mice is no longer recommended by either OIE or WHO. The rapid fluorescent focus inhibition test (RFFIT) has become the test of choice in most modern laboratories. Fluorescent antibody virus neutralisation (FAVN) test and ELISA have also been developed to measure the antirabies antibody titres in the vaccinated subjects (OIE Terrestrial Manual 2011; WHO 2012).

4.3.2.2 Rapid Fluorescent Focus Inhibition Test (RFFIT)

RFFIT is a serum neutralisation test which determines the rabies virus-neutralising antibody in the serum. It is a prescribed test for international trade. Challenge virus standard (CVS) strain CVS-11 and BHK-21 cells or mouse neuroblastoma cells are used to conduct the test (Meslin et al. 1996; OIE Terrestrial Manual 2011). Serial dilutions of serum are mixed with a standard amount of live rabies virus and incubated. The rabies virus-neutralising antibodies present in the serum neutralise the virus. Tissue culture cells are then added and incubated. The rabies virus which has not been neutralised by the antibody in the serum will infect the cells, which can be microscopically examined. Antibody titre in the serum can thus be calculated.

4.3.2.3 Fluorescent Antibody Virus Neutralisation (FAVN) Test

FAVN test is a virus neutralisation assay in cell culture that measures the response of an animal's immune system to the rabies vaccine. The test has been developed to screen animal sera by a standard method for an adequate level of rabies antibodies following vaccination. It is a prescribed test for international trade and is required by many rabies-free countries or regions for dogs and cats in order to qualify for a reduced quarantine period prior to entry. The test involves in vitro neutralisation of a constant amount of rabies virus (CVS strain adapted to cell culture) and then inoculating into the cell culture. Microplates are used to carry out the test (OIE Terrestrial Manual 2011). One plate is used for the titration of the CVS and for the controls that include OIE standard serum (0.5 IU/ml), naive dog serum (negative), and positive control or WHO standard serum. The other plates are used for the sera to be tested. The serial dilutions of the sera are titrated against CVS. After attempting neutralisation of virus, BHK-21 cells are added to detect the presence of non-neutralised virus. The plates after incubation are fixed and stained with FITC antirabies conjugate and examined for fluorescent cells. The serum titre is the dilution at which 100 % of the virus is neutralised in 50 % of the wells. This titre is expressed in IU/ml by comparing it with the neutralising dilution of the OIE serum of dog origin under the same experimental conditions.

4.3.2.4 Enzyme-Linked Immunosorbent Assay (ELISA)

The ELISA provides a rapid test that avoids the requirement to handle live rabies virus. Commercial indirect ELISA kits are available that allow detection of rabies antibodies in individuals and animals following vaccination (OIE Terrestrial Manual 2011). Serial dilutions of test sera and the control sera are placed in the wells of the microtitre ELISA plates precoated with the antigen. If rabies antibodies are present in the sera, they bind with the virus antigen fixed on the plate. Horseradish peroxidase conjugate is then added which binds with the retained antibody. After adequate incubation, the reaction is stopped by adding the stopping solution. The immobilised enzyme on the complexes can be quantified by spectrometric readings at 492 nm. Comparison of the readings of the test samples with that of the control sera provides the titre of antibodies in the test sera specimens.

It is a prescribed test for international trade. The test can be useful when facilities for RFFIT or FAVN are not available, as is usually the case in developing countries (WHO 2005).

References

CDC (2012) Rabies. Centers for Disease Control and Prevention. http://www.cdc.gov/rabies/. Accessed 30 Mar 2012

CFSPH (2009) Rabies. The Center for Food Security and Public Health, Iowa State University, Iowa. http://www.cfsph.iastate.edu/Factsheets/pdfs/rabies.pdf. Accessed 15 Mar 2011

Green SL, Smith L, Vernau W, Beacock SB (1992) Rabies in horses: 21 cases (1970–1990). J Am Vet Med Assoc 200:1133–1137

Hudson LC, Weinstock D, Jordan T, Bold-Fletcher NO (1996a) Clinical presentation of experimentally induced rabies in horses. Zentralbl Veterinarmed B 43:277–285

Hudson LC, Weinstock D, Jordan T, Bold-Fletcher NO (1996b) Clinical presentation of experimentally induced rabies in cattle and sheep. Zentralbl Veterinarmed B 43:85–95

Lembo T, Niezgoda M, Velasco-Villa A, Cleaveland S, Ernest E, Rupprecht CE (2006) Evaluation of a direct, rapid immunohistochemical test for rabies diagnosis. Emerg Infect Dis 12(2):310–313

Meslin FX, Kaplan MM, Koprowski H (1996) Laboratory techniques in rabies, 4th edn. World Health Organization, Geneva

Niezgoda M, Rupprecht CE (2006) Standard operating procedure for the direct rapid immunohistochemistry test for the detection of rabies virus antigen. National Laboratory Training Network Course, US Department of Health and Human Services. Centers for Disease Control and Prevention, Atlanta, pp 1–16

OIE Terrestrial Manual (2011) Manual of diagnostic tests and vaccines for terrestrial animals 2011. Chapter 2.1.13. Rabies. World Organisation for Animal Health. http://www.oie.int/international-standard-setting/terrestrial-manual/access-online/. Accessed 31 Mar 2012

Radostits OM, Gay CC, Hinchcliff KW, Constable PD (2007) Veterinary medicine – a textbook of the diseases of cattle, horses, sheep, pigs and goats, 10th edn. Saunders-Elsevier, Edinburgh

Shultz J (2004) Rabies. In: Shultz J (ed) Best practices for nuisance wildlife control operators: a training manual. New York State Department of Environmental Conservation, New York. http://www.nwco.net/PDF/whole_book.pdf. Accessed 18 Jan 2011

WHO (2005) WHO expert consultation on rabies. First report. WHO technical report series, no. 931. World Health Organization, Geneva

WHO (2010) Rabies vaccines: WHO position paper. Wkly Epidemiol Rec No 32 85:309–320

WHO (2012) Rabies. World Health Organization. www.who.int. Accessed 10 Mar 2012

5 Risk Assessment and Management of Exposures

Abstract

The assessment of risk of rabies transmission in individual cases is important in arriving at appropriate decision regarding the course of postexposure prophylaxis (PEP) requirements. The World Health Organization has laid down guidelines for differentiating the categories of potential rabies exposure and taking appropriate prophylactic measures. Development of a decision tree assists in risk evaluation. A three-pronged strategy is adopted to manage the exposures. It involves bite wound management, postexposure passive immunisation through rabies immunoglobulin (RIG), and vaccination for active immunity. Wound treatment includes mechanical and chemical action against rabies virus. RIG neutralises and destroys the virus while postexposure antirabies vaccination helps in developing active immunity against rabies. Pre-exposure prophylactic vaccination is also recommended in high-risk individuals. Intradermal rabies vaccination has emerged as a less expensive alternative to intramuscular route of vaccine administration. PEP treatment is a proven method of rabies prevention; however, prophylaxis failures and rabies-related deaths are encountered largely due to deviations from the recommended guidelines. There is no specific treatment after the onset of symptoms of rabies.

5.1 Human Exposure-Risk Assessment

Since the nature of bite or contact differs in each event and the epidemiology of rabies varies too in different regions, the assessment of risk of rabies transmission in individual cases is important in arriving at appropriate decision regarding the course of postexposure prophylaxis (PEP) requirement. Collection of detailed and accurate history of the exposure is essential for the risk assessment (Fig. 5.1).

A number of factors should be considered to assess the risk of exposure and take up appropriate prophylactic measures in individual cases as outlined by several public health organisations (NICD 2007; Georgia Department of Community Health 2011; Florida Department of Health 2012). These factors are briefly discussed below.

S.R. Garg, *Rabies in Man and Animals*, DOI 10.1007/978-81-322-1605-6_5,

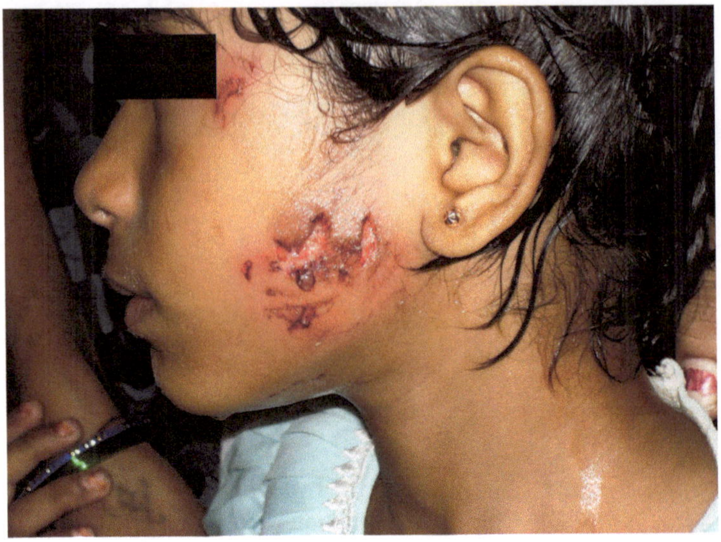

Fig. 5.1 A child with severe dog bite (Photo credit: Dr. B. J. Mahendra)

Table 5.1 The WHO guidelines for postexposure prophylactic measures (WHO 2010a)

Category	Type of exposure	Postexposure prophylactic recommendations
I	Touching or feeding animals, licks on intact skin (that is, no exposure)	No prophylaxis is required
II	Nibbling of uncovered skin, minor scratches, or abrasions without bleeding	Thorough washing and flushing of bite wounds and scratches for about 15 min with soap or detergent and copious amounts of water immediately or as early as possible
		Application of iodine-containing or similar viricidal topical preparation to wounds
		Immediate postexposure antirabies vaccination; PEP may be discontinued if the suspect animal is proved by appropriate laboratory examination to be free of rabies or, in the case of domestic dogs, cats, or ferrets, the animal remains healthy throughout a 10-day observation period starting from the date of the bite
III	Single or multiple transdermal bites or scratches, contamination of mucous membrane with saliva from licks, licks on broken skin, exposures to bats	Thorough washing and flushing of bite wounds and scratches for about 15 min with soap or detergent and copious amounts of water immediately or as early as possible
		Application of iodine-containing or similar viricidal topical preparation to wounds
		Immediate vaccination and administration of rabies immunoglobulin (RIG); PEP may be discontinued if the suspect animal is proved by appropriate laboratory examination to be free of rabies or, in the case of domestic dogs, cats, or ferrets, the animal remains healthy throughout a 10-day observation period starting from the date of the bite

5.1.1 Type of Exposure

The World Health Organization (WHO) has laid down guidelines for differentiating the potential rabies exposure into Category I, II, or III exposures based on the type of exposure (WHO 2010a). Appropriate prophylactic measures have also been recommended in different categories as shown in Table 5.1.

5.1.2 Type of Animal Leading to Exposure

The likelihood of rabies in different species of animals varies by region. In India and many other developing countries, dogs and cats remain the major reservoir and vector of rabies and represent an increased risk for rabies exposure. In such countries, free-roaming animals pose greater risk than those living in homes under supervision and their movements are restrained. On the other hand, the picture in many developed nations may be quite different because dogs and cats are less likely to become infected with rabies due to strict surveillance and regular updating of vaccination status in these animals. In these countries, the highest risk of rabies transmission is generally associated with bite exposure from terrestrial wild carnivores or bats. Although all species of livestock are susceptible to rabies, they may not be as frequently involved in inflicting bites to humans. Small rodents (squirrels, hamsters, guinea pigs, gerbils, chipmunks, rats, and mice) and lagomorphs (rabbits and hares) are rarely infected with rabies and have not been known to transmit rabies to humans and seldom require treatment.

5.1.3 Geographical Location of the Incident

Information regarding the endemicity of disease in the region of the exposure event can provide useful guidance regarding the PEP requirement. In rabies-endemic country like India, where every animal bite is potentially suspected as a rabid animal bite, the treatment should be started immediately.

5.1.4 Animal Behaviour and Health

Animal behaviour and its health status provide clue to the rabid disposition of the biting animal. Any animal, wild, domestic, caged, or feral, that shows signs of rabies typical to that species should be considered possibly rabid. Most free-ranging wild animals that normally avoid humans approaching or attacking humans or their pets should be considered possibly rabid.

5.1.5 Vaccination Status of the Biting Animal

Although unvaccinated animals are more likely to transmit rabies, vaccinated animals may also not be regarded as free from the risk of transmitting the infection. This is particularly so in the developing countries where critical rabies surveillance systems are generally not available. Many times the information about the pre-exposure prophylactic vaccination status of the implicated animal may not be reliable, the vaccination records may not be available, and the booster doses of rabies vaccination might not be current. In addition to it, evaluation of the post-vaccination immune status of vaccinated animals is usually impracticable in the developing countries. The vaccination of the biting animal might also be ineffective due to reasons such as improper administration, poor quality of vaccine, and poor health status of the animal. Due to these reasons and that a single shot of vaccine does not provide long-lasting protection against infection, a history of rabies vaccination in an animal is not always a guarantee that the biting animal is not rabid. Under such situations, it may not be advisable to withhold postexposure vaccination even if the animal is vaccinated (WHO 2010a); however, in developed countries, a currently vaccinated pet dog or cat may be unlikely to become infected with rabies.

5.1.6 Type of Encounter-Provoked Versus Unprovoked Bites

An unprovoked attack by an animal may be more likely than a provoked attack to indicate that the animal is rabid. Provoked attacks or bites by domestic dogs and cats may be the sequelae of certain circumstances created by any person even though the animal might not be rabid. Though it may be difficult to distinguish the provoked attacks from the unprovoked ones, but certain circumstances at the time of attacks may help in assessing the risk as listed below (CDCB 2012). However, whether a bite was provoked rather than unprovoked should not be considered a guarantee that the animal is not rabid as it can be difficult to understand and pinpoint the cause of provocation for an attack. Any bite from a high-risk species, whether provoked or unprovoked, should be considered a rabies exposure unless proven otherwise by laboratory testing of the animal or observation for 10 days in case of dogs and cats.

5.1.6.1 Signs of Provoked Attack

- Entering an unfamiliar compound which is guarded by a dog
- Threatening or injuring the animal or the pet owner
- Beating an animal
- Playing in an area where a dog is located
- Petting or playing with a strange dog
- Walking past a dog
- Stepping on or bumping into a dog
- Stepping on a cat
- Interfering in a dog fight
- Taking puppies from their mother
- Disturbing the animal's offspring
- Disturbing the animal while eating
- Handling or removing the animal's food
- Handling/startling a sleeping animal
- Invading the animal's living space
- Restraining or handling sick or injured animals
- Attempting to feed or handle an apparently healthy but unfamiliar domestic animal

5.1.6.2 Unprovoked Attack

- Attack by a dog for an unknown reason and from an unknown site
- Biting by the victim's own dog without such prior history of aggressive behaviour

5.1.7 Observational and Laboratory Findings on Animal's Rabies Status

Pet dogs, cats, and livestock can be isolated and observed to determine their rabies status after exposing a person to rabies. However, feral or unidentified dogs and cats may not be available for either observation or testing. Animals killed during attacks, euthanised, or dying after capture should be tested as soon as possible to decide about the initiation and continuation of PEP administration. The PEP immunisation should be started immediately after the bite unless the biting animal is proved to be not rabid. The treatment may be modified if the biting animal (dog or cat) remains healthy throughout the observation period of 10 days by converting PEP to pre-exposure vaccination by skipping the vaccine dose on day 14 and administering it on day 28 while using the Essen Schedule. The observation period is valid for dogs and cats only. The natural history of rabies in mammals other than dogs or cats is not fully understood and therefore the 10-day observation period may not be applicable.

5.1.8 Bite by Wild Animals

Bite by all wild animals should be treated as Category III exposure regardless of the animal's health status or behaviour as it may be difficult to reliably interpret the clinical signs of rabies among wildlife. Moreover, these animals have been shown to sometimes have virus in their saliva for a week or more before becoming apparently ill or showing reliable signs of the disease. Some of these animals may belong to a species known for its status as a rabies reservoir or in which rabies is diagnosed frequently. All bites by such wildlife, therefore, must be considered possible exposures to the rabies virus. PEP should be initiated as soon as possible unless the animal is available for testing and it is proved to be negative for rabies.

5.1.9 Bat Rabies

Bat rabies has not been conclusively proven in India; hence exposure to bats may not warrant treatment in the country (NICD 2007). However, in all those parts of the world where bat rabies is prevalent or bats are implicated as reservoirs for rabies, rabies PEP is recommended for all persons with bite, scratch, or mucous membrane exposure to a bat, unless the bat is available for testing and shows no evidence of rabies. PEP might also be appropriate even if a bite, scratch, or mucous membrane exposure is not apparent but when there is reasonable probability that such exposure might have occurred.

5.1.10 Patient's Previous Immunisation Status

The individuals who are not previously immunised against rabies are at much greater risk and require complete course of PEP immunisation according to the exposure-risk category requirements. However, the persons who are previously immunised against rabies through pre-exposure vaccination with modern cell culture vaccine may require less number (two) of doses of antirabies vaccine and may not require RIG at all. On rare occasions, it may be required to evaluate the immune status of the person in the laboratory.

5.1.11 Human-to-Human Transmission

The risk of rabies transmission to other humans from a human rabies case is very minimal, and there has never been a well-documented case of human-to-human transmission, other than the few cases resulting from organ transplant. However, people who have been exposed closely to the secretions of a patient with rabies may be offered PEP as a precautionary measure (NICD 2007).

5.2 Human Exposure Management

A person after exposure to infection through animal bite or contact with a rabid or suspected animal or infected material should be handled with utmost speed to prevent the disease. Three-pronged strategy is adopted that involves the management of bite wound and PEP immunisation against rabies as shown below.

- Step 1. Bite wound management
- Step 2. Postexposure passive immunisation with RIG where necessary
- Step 3. Postexposure vaccination for active immunity

Development of a decision tree assists in the evaluation of the rabies transmission risk associated with an animal bite and in taking correct decision regarding the need of PEP immunisation and the regimen to be adopted in each case of exposure. Decision trees are evolved taking into consideration the epidemiological features of the disease in a geographical area and the extent of risk posed by different species of animals in that area. The availability of rapid diagnostic facilities may also be a factor in a decision tree algorithm. A decision tree prepared by the National Centre for Disease Control (previously National Institute of Communicable Diseases) to provide guidance on human rabies prophylaxis in India is shown in Fig. 5.2 (NICD 2007).

5.2.1 Bite Wound Management

The best way to ward off the exposure to rabies virus is to avoid bites and licking of fresh wounds or mucous membranes by the mammals, mainly dogs, monkeys, bats, cats, and wild animals. However, when such exposures take place, immediate medical care is critical. As the rabies virus enters the body through a bite or scratch, it is important to remove as much saliva, and thereby the virus, from the wound as is possible by efficient wound cleansing without causing additional trauma. Prompt wound care can substantially reduce the risk of infection.

For Category II and III exposures, this should be done by prompt and gentle thorough washing and flushing of the wound for about 15 min with soap or detergent and copious amount of running water. If soap and detergent are not immediately available, washing with running water alone is also useful. After thorough washing and drying the wound, disinfection of the wound should be carried out with ethanol (700 ml/l) or iodine

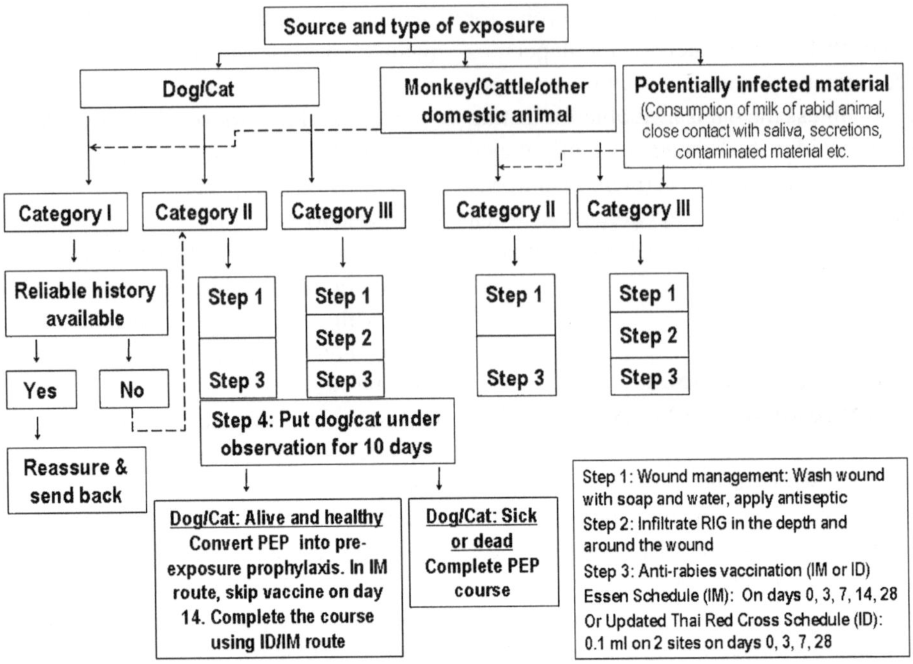

Fig. 5.2 Decision tree: guide to postexposure prophylaxis in India (Adapted from NICD 2007)

(tincture or aqueous solution), povidone iodine, or similarly viricidal topical preparation (NICD 2007; WHO 2010a, b). Antiseptic agents such as Betadine, alcohol, chloroxylenol (Dettol), chlorhexidine gluconate, and cetrimide solution (Savlon) may be applied in appropriate recommended concentration. Rabies virus can be inactivated by soap solutions, 45–75 % ethanol, iodine preparations, quaternary ammonium compounds, or a low pH. Being susceptible to ultraviolet radiation, the virus is rapidly inactivated in sunlight. Proper care of wound removes or reduces the virus and lowers the risk of rabies to the extent of 50–70 %.

Substances like turmeric, *neem*, chilli, lime, salt, oil, plant extracts, and coffee powder should not be applied on the wound. These irritants may propel the virus deep into the wound causing nerve infection. In case such irritants have been applied on the wound at home, the extraneous material especially oil should be removed by washing the wound with soap or detergent and flushing the wound with copious amount of water immediately.

The wound washing is most effective when fresh wound is cleaned immediately but it should be carried out even at a later stage if the patient reports for treatment late and the wound is unhealed that can be washed. As rabies virus can persist and even multiply at the site of bite for a long time, wound cleaning after a delay will also be useful.

Bandaging, dressing, and suturing of wounds should be avoided; these should be left open without suturing for a few days. However, if surgically suturing is necessary to control the bleeding or for functional or cosmetic reasons, RIG should be administered into the wound before closing the wound and loose sutures should be applied. The use of local anaesthetic is not contraindicated in wound management.

Cauterisation of wound is no longer recommended as it leaves very bad scar and does not confer any additional advantage over washing the wound with water and soap. Tetanus toxoid should be injected to unimmunised individuals. A suitable course of an antibiotic may be recommended to prevent the wound sepsis.

5.2.2 Postexposure Prophylactic (PEP) Immunisation

Wound treatment includes mechanical and chemical action only against rabies virus. It should always be followed by exposure-risk assessment by the healthcare specialist and adequate PEP immunisation where required. Antirabies immunisation neutralises and destroys the virus. It should be initiated immediately following a transdermal bite or scratch by an animal suspected of being rabid or when possibly infectious material, usually saliva, comes into direct contact with the victim's mucosa or with fresh skin wounds according to the WHO guidelines (WHO 2010a, 2012).

Postexposure antirabies immunisation involves administration of antirabies vaccine with or without application of RIG based on the category of exposure as shown in Table 5.1.

PEP should start immediately wherever recommended according to the guidelines. The persons who present for evaluation and rabies PEP even months after having been bitten should be dealt with in the same manner as if the contact occurred recently. Pregnancy and infancy are never contraindications to PEP (WHO 2010b). Apart from the category of exposure, factors such as the epidemiological likelihood of the implicated animal being rabid, clinical features of the animal, and its availability for observation and laboratory testing should be taken into consideration when deciding whether to initiate PEP. If the animal inflicting the wound is suspected of being rabid and is not apprehended, PEP should be instituted immediately (WHO 2012).

The institution of PEP in the exposed individuals should not be postponed awaiting the results of laboratory diagnosis because in many cases it may delay the immunisation process, jeopardising its success. Many times, particularly in developing countries, the information about the pre-exposure prophylactic vaccination status of the implicated animal may not be reliable; hence it may not be advisable to withhold the postexposure vaccination even if the animal is vaccinated. Similarly, in certain situations where a reliable history cannot be obtained, the cases may be treated as Category II or III, particularly in rabies-enzootic areas, even though the animal is considered to be healthy at the time of exposure (WHO 2010a, 2012).

PEP treatment should be continued until a clear and unequivocal negative laboratory report is provided. A positive test by any one of several recognised procedures overrides negative reactions in the others. Where a doubtful result is obtained in any single test, recourse to the other tests available is essential in order to arrive at a definitive conclusion. PEP may be terminated or modified at that point if the animal involved is a dog or cat that remains healthy for an observation period of 10 days after the exposure occurred; or if the animal is humanely killed and proven to be negative for rabies by a reliable diagnostic laboratory using a prescribed test (WHO 2010a, b, 2012). However, the circumstances may occasionally justify the initiation or continuation of treatment by the physician, e.g. suspicious clinical signs in the animal, or an attack in a rabies-enzootic area by an animal that could not be caught or killed for laboratory diagnosis. In areas where canine or wildlife rabies is enzootic, adequate laboratory surveillance is in place, and data from laboratory and field experience indicate that there is no infection in the species involved, local health authorities may not recommend antirabies prophylaxis (WHO 2010a, b, 2012).

5.2.3 Administration of Postexposure Antirabies Vaccine

After an exposure or suspected exposure to rabies, active immunisation is achieved by administration of safe and potent cell culture vaccines. Postexposure antirabies vaccination should start immediately wherever recommended according to the guidelines. All patients with Category II and III exposures require PEP vaccination. In addition to it, administration of RIG is required in all Category III exposures and in those Category II exposures that involve immunodeficient people. Due to the serious implications of the rabies exposure, vaccination should not be delayed or deferred.

5.2.3.1 Antirabies Vaccines

The vaccination should be done using vaccine regimens and routes of administration that have been proven to be safe and effective (WHO 2010b). All cell culture vaccines should comply with the WHO-recommended potency of ≥2.5 IU per single intramuscular dose. The WHO strongly advocates the use of purified rabies vaccines prepared on cell culture or embryonated eggs for PEP that comply with the WHO criteria for potency and innocuity and have been assessed satisfactorily in humans in well-designed field trials. Cell culture vaccines have proven to be safe and effective in preventing rabies. Purified vaccines do not have contraindication.

In India, modern cell culture vaccines are used. Due to the reactogenic nature of the nervous tissue vaccine, its use has been completely stopped and its production was discontinued in the country in the year 2004 (NICD 2007).

5.2.3.2 Vaccine Administration Routes, Sites, and Dose

The postexposure vaccination involves injecting vaccines through intramuscular route according to an approved vaccination regimen. The dose of the vaccine is usually 1 ml or 0.5 ml depending on the type of vaccine. All intramuscular injections must be given into the deltoid region or, in small children, into the anterolateral area of the thigh. Vaccine should never be administered in the gluteal region because the fat present in this region retards the absorption of antigen and hence impairs the generation of optimal immune response (NICD 2007; WHO 2010a, 2012).

In order to reduce the cost of PEP vaccination, intradermal administration of vaccine has also been recommended in which less volume of vaccine is required. Wherever approved, it involves multisite intradermal inoculation of 0.1 ml vaccine per site (deltoid and thigh regions) according to an approved regimen (NICD 2007; WHO 2010a, 2012).

5.2.3.3 Vaccination Regimen for Intramuscular Administration

Two regimens of PEP vaccination through intramuscular route have been recommended by the WHO. One of these is a 5-dose schedule, while another is a 4-dose schedule (WHO 2010a, 2012). The day of administration of the first dose should be taken as day 0 in cases where the vaccination could not be initiated on the day of bite itself.

i. **The 5-dose regimen**. It consists of a 5-dose schedule. One dose of the vaccine is administered each on days 0, 3, 7, 14, and 28 intramuscularly in the deltoid muscle or anterolateral thigh muscle. This vaccination schedule involves five visits of the patient to the healthcare facility. It is also known as Essen regimen.
ii. **The 4-dose regimen**. This abbreviated multisite schedule, the 2-1-1 regimen, prescribes two doses on day 0, followed by one dose each on day 7 and day 21. On day 0, one dose is given in the deltoid muscle of the right arm and one dose in the left arm. Subsequently, one dose each is applied on day 7 and day 21 in the deltoid muscle. This vaccination schedule is also known as Zagreb regimen. It involves only three visits of the patient for vaccination which may be helpful in cases where the patient has to travel and is unable to make five visits to the healthcare centre for vaccination.

An alternative reduced (4-dose) PEP regimen has been recommended by the United States Advisory Committee on Immunization Practices (ACIP) for healthy, fully immunocompetent, exposed people who receive wound care plus high-quality RIG plus the WHO-prequalified rabies vaccines. It consists of 4 doses administered intramuscularly on days 0, 3, 7, and 14 (Rupprecht et al. 2009; WHO 2010a, 2012). Previously, ACIP recommended a 5-dose rabies vaccination regimen with human diploid cell vaccine (HDCV) or purified chick embryo cell vaccine (PCECV). These new recommendations reduce the number of vaccine doses to four. The reduction in doses recommended for PEP was based in part on evidence from rabies virus pathogenesis data, experimental animal work, clinical studies, and epidemiological surveillance. These studies indicated that four vaccine doses in combination with RIG elicited adequate immune responses and that a fifth dose of vaccine did not contribute to more favourable outcomes (CDC 2010b). It has been inferred that the administration of only 4 doses of vaccine during prophylaxis on days 0, 3, 7, and 14 will induce an adequate, long-lasting immune response that is able to neutralise rabies virus and prevent disease in all patients when applied appropriately with proper wound care and immunoglobulin (Rupprecht et al. 2009).

5.2.3.4 Vaccination Regimen for Intramuscular Administration in India

The Essen regimen is the currently approved regimen for intramuscular administration of rabies PEP cell culture vaccines in India. The course for PEP consists of five injections on days 0, 3, 7, 14, and 28. The sixth injection on day 90 should be considered as optional and should be given to those individuals who are immunologically deficient or those at the extremes of age and on steroid therapy. Day 0 indicates the date of first injection (NICD 2007).

5.2.3.5 Vaccines and Regimen Approved for Intradermal Administration

The WHO prescribes the 2-site regimen for intradermal administration of a vaccine approved for intradermal use. In this method, two doses of vaccine (0.1 ml each) are injected at two sites (one in each of the upper arm) on days 0, 3, 7, and 28. This regimen can be used for people with Category II and Category III exposures in countries where the intradermal route has been endorsed by national health authorities. Only vaccines that have been demonstrated to be safe and efficacious should be used by the intradermal route. The vaccines and brands approved by WHO (2012) for this purpose include purified Vero cell rabies vaccine (PVRV) (Verorab™, Imovax™, Rabies vero™, TRC Verorab™) and PCECV (Rabipur™).

5.2.3.6 Vaccines and Regimen Approved for Intradermal Administration in India

Considering the WHO recommendations and the results of safety, efficacy, and feasibility trials conducted in India, the Drug Controller General of India (DCGI) has approved the use of intradermal vaccination regimen for rabies PEP vaccination according to the prescribed guidelines. The following vaccines and brands have been approved by DCGI for use by intradermal route in the country (NICD 2007):

1. Verorab (PVRV), Aventis Pasteur (Sanofi Pasteur) India Pvt. Ltd.
2. Rabipur (PCECV), Chiron Behring Vaccines Pvt. Ltd.
3. PVRV, Pasteur Institute of India, Coonoor
4. Abhayrab (PVRV), Human Biologicals Institute

The Updated Thai Red Cross Schedule (2-2-2-0-2) is the approved vaccination regimen in India. It involves injection of 0.1 ml of reconstituted vaccine per intradermal site and on two such sites per visit (one on each deltoid area, an inch above the insertion of deltoid muscle) on days 0, 3, 7, and 28. The day 0 is the day of administration of first dose of intradermal rabies vaccine and may not be the day of rabies exposure/animal bite.

5.2.3.7 Postexposure Prophylaxis of Previously Immunised Persons

For rabies-exposed patients who have previously undergone complete postexposure treatment or those who can document previous complete pre-exposure vaccination with a cell culture vaccine, only two intramuscular or intradermal doses of a cell culture vaccine, one on day 0 and another on day 3, are sufficient. Authentic records of previous immunisations are very important for making correct decisions in such cases. This regimen also applies to the people vaccinated against rabies who have demonstrated rabies virus-neutralising antibody titres of ≥0.5 IU/ml. Administration of RIG is not necessary in such cases (WHO 2010a, 2012).

As an alternative to this regimen, the patient may be offered a single-visit 4-site intradermal regimen consisting of four injections of 0.1 ml equally distributed over left and right deltoids and thighs (WHO 2010a, 2012).

Full course of PEP vaccination should be given to those persons who previously received pre-exposure or postexposure prophylaxis with vaccines of unproven potency. Thus, persons who have previously received full postexposure treatment with nervous tissue vaccine should be treated as fresh case and may be given treatment accordingly. Similarly, those patients in whom immunological memory is no longer assured due to immunosuppressive causes should be given complete PEP vaccination (NICD 2007; WHO 2010b).

5.2.3.8 Postexposure Prophylaxis of Immunodeficient Persons

Several studies of patients with HIV/AIDS (immunodeficient disposition) have reported that those with low CD4 (<200 counts) will mount a significantly lower or no detectable neutralising antibody response to rabies vaccination. Consequently, in immunocompromised individuals including patients with HIV/AIDS, a complete series of five doses of intramuscular cell culture vaccine in combination with comprehensive wound management and local infiltration with RIG is required for patients with Category II and III exposures. When feasible, the rabies virus-neutralising antibody response should be determined 2–4 weeks following vaccination to assess the possible need for an additional dose of the vaccine. An antibody titre of 0.5 IU/ml or more in serum as measured by the rapid fluorescent focus inhibition test (RFFIT) or the fluorescent antibody virus neutralisation (FAVN) test is considered as protective (WHO 2010a).

5.2.3.9 Contraindications

For PEP vaccination there are no contraindications as it is a life-saving procedure. Rabies being a fatal disease, PEP vaccination takes preference over any other consideration. Pregnancy, lactation, infancy, old age, and concurrent illness are not contraindications. The immune response to rabies vaccine in infants and the elderly, without specific immunosuppressive conditions, is reported to be adequate. Vaccination is immunogenic, safe, and highly efficacious in pregnant women (WHO 2005). No reported risk of abortion or other harm to the foetus has been reported due to administration of PEP vaccination with cell culture vaccines in pregnant women (Sudarshan et al. 2007; Abazeed and Cinti 2007). Rabies PEP should never be withheld from pregnant women as it is a life-saving vaccine. This is also the case for PEP in immunocompromised individuals, including children with HIV/AIDS (Thisyakorn et al. 2000).

People taking chloroquine for malaria treatment or prophylaxis may have a reduced response to intradermal rabies vaccination (IDRV). For this reason, vaccine should be administered to this group of patients by intramuscular route (Bernard et al. 1985; Pappaioanou et al. 1986; WHO 2005).

5.2.3.10 Precautions

Apart from choosing appropriate vaccine, regimen, injection site, and route of administration, care should be taken regarding storage, transportation, reconstitution, and handling of the vaccine. Most cell culture vaccines are marketed in freeze-dried (lyophilised) form, which is more tolerant of temperature fluctuations, but it is recommended that these vaccines should be kept and transported at a temperature range of 2–8 °C. Freezing does not damage the lyophilised vaccine but there are chances of breakage of ampoule containing the diluent. Liquid vaccines should never be frozen. The lyophilised vaccine should be reconstituted with the diluent provided with the vaccine immediately prior to use. However, in case of unforeseen delay it should not be used after 6–8 h of reconstitution (NICD 2007).

5.2.3.11 Side Effects

Cell culture vaccines are widely accepted as safe, well tolerated, and least reactogenic. However, minor and transient erythema, pain, and/or swelling may occur at the site of injection in 35–45 % of vaccinees, particularly following intradermal administration of a booster (Dreesen et al. 1986; Fishbein et al. 1989; Briggs et al. 2000). Mild systemic adverse events following immunisation, such as transient fever, headache, dizziness, and gastrointestinal symptoms, have been observed in 5–15 % of vaccinees (Fishbein et al. 1989; Lang et al. 1998; Quiambao et al. 2005). Serious adverse events mainly of allergic or neurological nature rarely occur (Dobardzic et al. 2007; WHO 2010a).

5.2.3.12 Discontinuation of Vaccination

PEP may be discontinued if the suspect animal is proved by appropriate laboratory examination to be free of rabies or, in the case of domestic dogs, cats, or ferrets, the animal remains healthy throughout a 10-day observation period starting from the date of the bite (WHO 2010a).

5.2.3.13 Switch Over from One Type/ Brand of Vaccine to Another

It would be better to use the same vaccine in all doses in a case. Switching over from one type/ brand of cell culture vaccine to another type/ brand should be avoided, but when it is not possible to complete a full course with the same vaccine, another type of WHO-recommended cell culture vaccine should be used to complete the PEP (NICD 2007; WHO 2010a).

5.2.3.14 Switch Over from One Route of Vaccination to Another

The effect of change of the route of vaccine administration (e.g. from intramuscular to intradermal) during PEP on vaccine immunogenicity has so far not been examined. The practice of switch over to different route midway the course of PEP vaccination should be the exception (WHO 2010b).

5.2.4 Application of Rabies Immunoglobulin (RIG)

The objective of the PEP is to neutralise and destroy rabies virus that was inoculated into a victim's body at the time of exposure. It is, therefore, essential that neutralising antibody directed against rabies virus is produced as early as possible. However, primary vaccination takes 7–14 days to produce protective antibody titre. Thus, a victim may remain vulnerable to rabies during the initial period after exposure. Because rabies is invariably fatal, the administration of RIG provides instant passive immunity early in the vaccination regimen. Administration of RIG into a bite wound delivers ready-made antirabies antibodies specifically targeted against rabies virus to the anatomical region where the virus was injected during the exposure (WHO 2011). RIG has the property of binding with the rabies virus, thereby causing its neutralisation and thus preventing it from entering the nerve cells. However, in common practice, it has been observed that administration of RIG in bite cases is almost ignored, particularly in the developing countries due to ignorance or unavailability of RIG.

Administration of RIG side by side with antirabies vaccine is the best specific systemic treatment available for PEP of rabies in humans, although experience indicated that vaccine alone was sufficient for minor (Category II) exposures in immunocompetent people (WHO 2012). According to the WHO guidelines, besides antirabies vaccine, RIG must be administered in all cases of Category III exposure and in the Category II exposures occurring in immunodeficient people. Failure to use RIG where indicated is one of the causes of failure of PEP. Care should be taken that RIG is not used alone without proper antirabies vaccination.

RIG for passive immunisation is administered only once, preferably at, or as soon as possible after, the initiation of postexposure vaccination. Administration of RIG beyond the seventh day after the first dose of antirabies vaccine is not indicated because an active antibody response to the cell culture vaccine is presumed to have occurred by that time and RIG may interfere with the vaccine-induced antibody production (WHO 2012).

5.2.4.1 Types of RIG

Two types of RIG, human RIG (HRIG) and equine RIG (ERIG), are available. HRIG has a relatively slow clearance (the half-life is about 21 days), so it is the preferred product, particularly in cases of multiple severe exposures and bites on the head, face, and hands. However, HRIG is generally in short supply and available mainly in industrialised countries. Where it is not available or affordable, equine immunoglobulin or F(ab′)2 products of equine immunoglobulin should be used. ERIG is raised by hyperimmunisation of horses. Because of its heterologous origin, ERIG carries a small risk of anaphylactic reaction

(1/45,000 cases). However, most of the currently manufactured ERIG preparations are highly purified, so the occurrence of adverse events has been significantly reduced. These are potent, safe, and considerably less expensive than HRIG. HRIG is free from the side effects encountered in a serum of heterologous origin (WHO 2010a, 2012).

5.2.4.2 Dose of RIG

The recommended dose of HRIG is 20 IU/kg bodyweight (total maximum 1,500 IU) and that of ERIG and F(ab´)2 products 40 IU/kg bodyweight (total maximum 3,000 IU). Because of longer half-life, HRIG is given in half the dose of ERIG. The total dose should not exceed the recommended levels as it may suppress the antibody production by the vaccine (NICD 2007; WHO 2010a, b).

5.2.4.3 Administration of RIG

RIG should be instilled carefully using 26 G needle into the depth of all wounds and also infiltrated around the wounds with least traumatisation. The full dose of RIG, or as much as is anatomically feasible, should be administered into and around the wound site. Any remaining RIG should be injected into the thigh region intramuscularly at a site distant from the vaccine administrative site. If the calculated dose and the resultant volume of RIG are too small, for example, as in case of a severely bitten child, it may be diluted two- to three-fold in sterile saline to infiltrate all wounds adequately. RIG should always be brought to room temperature (20–25 °C) before use, and it should never be administered in the same syringe or at the same anatomical site as vaccine (NICD 2007; WHO 2010a).

5.2.4.4 Precautions While Administering RIG

The Association for Prevention and Control of Rabies in India (APCRI) has published guidelines for the persons administering RIG (APCRI 2009). The APCRI recommends that the healthcare workers may observe the following precautions while administering RIG:

- The patient should not be on an empty stomach.
- The RIG vial(s) taken out from the refrigerator should be kept outside for a few minutes before administration to the patient to bring to room temperature/body temperature.
- While infiltrating RIG into bite wounds, care must be taken to avoid injecting into blood vessels and nerves. Sufficient care must also be taken while infiltrating RIG into bite wounds near the eyes and genital region. Anatomical feasibility should always be kept in mind while injecting RIG.
- While injecting into finger tips, care must be taken to avoid the compartment syndrome.
- All emergency drugs and facilities for managing any adverse reactions must be available.
- If ERIG is being administered, patient's history should be carefully taken regarding any previous administration of horse sera, viz. anti-tetanus, anti-diphtheria, anti-gas gangrene, anti-snake venom serum, and even anti-rabies sera (ERIG).
- The patient should be kept under observation for at least one hour after ERIG administration and then discharged (APCRI 2009).

5.2.4.5 Sensitivity Test Before Administration of ERIG

Because of the chances of anaphylactic shock due to administration of ERIG, sensitivity testing (skin test) is usually advised before giving ERIG. The skin test may be performed according to the instructions provided by the ERIG manufacturer. The test in general involves the following steps (NICD 2007; APCRI 2009):

- The patient is kept in a sitting position.
- The baseline pulse, blood pressure, and respiratory rate of the patient are recorded.
- 0.1 ml ERIG diluted 1:10 in physiological saline is injected intradermally into the flexor surface of the forearm to raise a bleb of about 3–4 mm diameter.
- Simultaneously, an equal amount of normal saline is injected as a negative control on the flexor surface of the other forearm (control injection).
- Constant watch is kept on the pulse, blood pressure, and respiratory rate of the patient for 15 min. The patient is also watched for any local or systemic reaction. After 15 min, the site of ERIG injection is observed for an

increase in diameter to >10 mm of induration surrounded by flare. The sign is taken as positive skin test, provided the reaction on the saline test on the other arm (control) was negative.
- An increase or abrupt fall in blood pressure, syncope, hurried breathing, palpitations, and any other systemic manifestations are taken as positive test.

The skin sensitivity test is considered negative when there is no reaction in both the forearms. If patient is sensitive to ERIG, HRIG should be used. It is important to note that a negative skin test must never reassure the physician that no anaphylactic reaction will occur. The skin testing may detect the rare case of IgE-mediated (type I) hypersensitivity to equine serum protein, but majority of reactions to ERIG result from complement activation and are not IgE-mediated and will not be predicted by skin testing (NICD 2007; APCRI 2009). However, the ERIG manufacturers generally recommend a compulsory skin test to check for hypersensitivity before the full dose administration of ERIG. In such circumstances, it is advisable to perform the skin sensitivity test to comply with the local drug laws and to avoid any subsequent litigation regarding medical negligence (APCRI 2009).

According to the WHO, there are no scientific grounds for performing a skin test prior to administering equine immunoglobulin because it may not predict reactions. Otherwise too, despite the probability of anaphylactic reaction, administration of immunoglobulin is essential whatever the results of skin test because of the life-threatening nature of rabies. Thus, the treating physician should be prepared to manage anaphylaxis which, though rare, could occur during any stage of administration irrespective of the outcome of the skin test (APCRI 2009; WHO 2010a, 2012).

5.2.4.6 Physician's Preparedness for Anaphylactic Reaction

The APCRI guidelines for persons administering RIG to manage a situation of anaphylactic reaction while administering ERIG are available (APCRI 2009). According to these guidelines, those administering ERIG should always be ready to treat anaphylactic reactions with injection of adrenaline, hydrocortisone hemisuccinate, pheniramine maleate, ranitidine, deriphyllin, and dopamine. Intravenous fluids and oxygen cylinder should be kept ready and used if needed. ERIG should preferably be given in a hospital facility under close medical supervision.

5.2.4.7 RIG Tolerance and Side Effects

With RIG, there may be transient tenderness at the injection site and a brief rise in body temperature, which do not require any treatment. Skin reactions are extremely rare. RIG is never to be given intravenously as this could produce symptoms of shock, especially in patients with antibody deficiency syndromes. Serum sickness occurs in 1–6 % of patients usually 7 to 10 days after injection of ERIG, but it has not been reported after treatment with HRIG (NICD 2007).

5.2.4.8 RIG Unavailability Situation

In circumstances where RIG is not available, greater emphasis should be given to proper wound toileting followed by Essen Schedule of cell culture vaccine with double dose on day 0 at 2 different sites intramuscularly (on 0 day: 2 doses on left and right deltoid, followed by single shot on 3, 7, 14, and 28 days). It is emphasised that doubling the first dose of vaccine is not a replacement to RIG. A full course of vaccine should follow (NICD 2007).

5.2.4.9 Delay in RIG Administration

If immunoglobulin was not administered when vaccination was begun, it can be administered up to the seventh day after the administration of the first dose of vaccine. RIG is not indicated beyond the seventh day, since an antibody response to antirabies vaccine is presumed to have occurred.

5.2.4.10 Current Scenario of RIG Administration

Despite the fact that effective PEP against rabies requires two-pronged strategy, i.e. active immunisation and passive immunisation, administration of RIG is commonly ignored in most cases, particularly in the developing countries, partly due to high cost or unavailability and partly due to ignorance. According to the WHO (2012), the current situation concerning passive immunisation in the developing countries is as shown below.

- Less than 1 % of all postexposure treatment are comprised of vaccine and serum.
- HRIG is not widely available and is too expensive for most people (about $250 per adult patient, approximately five times more expensive than purified horse serum).
- Cheaper and safe (purified pepsin digested horse serum) ERIG is available in limited quantities and in most situations is inaccessible to those that need it most.

As noted by the WHO (2012), this situation is getting worse due to the following circumstances:

- More and more international manufacturers are discontinuing ERIG production.
- Where production of purified equine products has been initiated (e.g. Thailand), it remains limited and hardly satisfies the national needs.
- Animal protection groups condemn and oppose the animal rearing for serum production.

5.3 Pre-exposure Antirabies Vaccination

Pre-exposure prophylactic vaccination is done to attain active immunity in high-risk individuals prior to a rabies exposure. It is recommended to those who are at continual, frequent, or increased risk of exposure to the rabies virus, either as a result of their residence or occupation (Fig. 5.3). Such individuals include veterinarians, animal handlers, dogcatchers, wildlife wardens, quarantine officers, laboratory workers dealing with rabies virus or other lyssaviruses or infected material, postmen, delivery personnel, pet owners, and schoolchildren. Travellers from rabies-free areas to rabies-endemic areas should also be vaccinated regardless of duration of stay (NICD 2007; WHO 2010a). Children in highly endemic areas may be considered if vaccine quantities are adequately available (WHO 2010b).

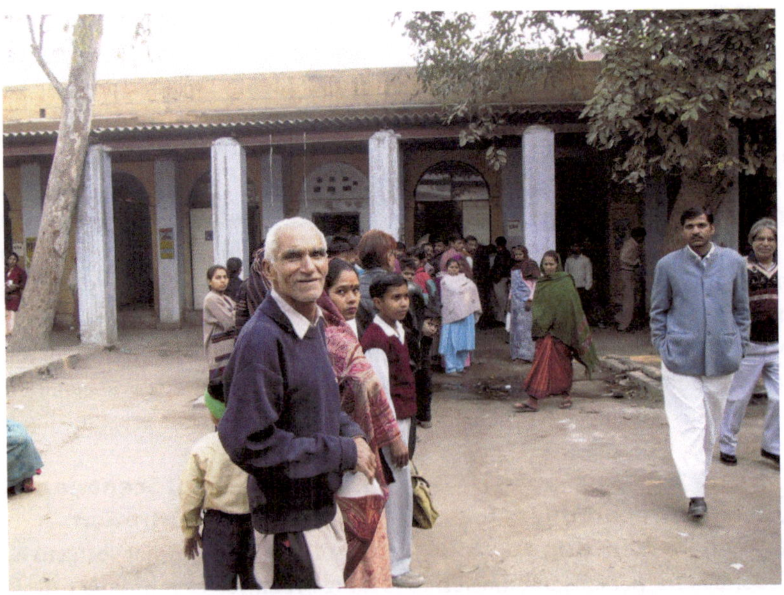

Fig. 5.3 People awaiting pre-exposure vaccination during rabies control programme (Photo courtesy: Dr. Deborrah Briggs)

5.3.1 Pre-exposure Vaccination Regimen

Same vaccines are used for pre-exposure prophylaxis as in case of PEP but the vaccination regimen is different. Pre-exposure vaccination requires invariably three doses of intramuscular vaccination on days 0, 7, and 21 or 28. Each dose consists of 1 ml or 0.5 ml vaccine (volume depending on the type of vaccine) injected in the deltoid area of the arm in adults and the children (above 2 years). For children aged less than 2 years, the anterolateral area of the thigh is recommended. Rabies vaccine should not be administered in the gluteal area, as the induction of an adequate immune response may be less reliable.

Intradermal administration of 0.1 ml volume on days 0, 7, and 21 or 28 is an acceptable alternative to the standard intramuscular route. It is important that enough number of individuals is available in one session of intradermal pre-exposure vaccination so that all opened vials are used within 6–8 h (WHO 2010a). Unutilised vials may lead to wastage of the vaccine and economic loss.

If antimalarial chemoprophylaxis is applied concurrently, intramuscular route is preferable to the intradermal route of injection (WHO 2010b).

5.3.2 Booster Dose Requirement

Periodic booster injections are recommended as an extra precaution only for people whose occupation puts them at continual or frequent risk of exposure. Because vaccine-induced immunity persists in most cases for years, a booster would be recommended only if rabies virus-neutralising antibody titres fall to <0.5 IU/ml. If the facilities are available, antibody monitoring of personnel at risk is preferred to the administration of routine boosters. For people who are potentially at risk of laboratory exposure to high concentrations of live rabies virus, antibody testing should be done every 6 months while those not at continual risk of exposure should have serological monitoring every 2 years (WHO 2010a). Such individuals on getting exposed to rabies virus after successful pre-exposure immunisation require only two booster injections of vaccine given on days 0 and 3 without any RIG.

5.4 Intradermal Rabies Vaccination (IDRV)

The full course of postexposure rabies vaccination by intramuscular route is quite expensive. The total cost of an average PEP course typically ranges between US$40 and US$49 in Africa and Asia as shown in studies. These estimates include the cost of biologicals and of their administration (materials for injection such as syringes, needles, and swabs and staff salaries) and patient's expenses towards transport to and from medical facilities and loss of income (Partners for Rabies Prevention 2010). The costs could even be much higher in certain settings. The high cost thus may limit the administration of cell culture vaccines in many areas, particularly in the developing countries, where canine rabies is widespread. Intradermal administration of these vaccines requires only 1–2 vials of vaccine to complete a full course of PEP, thereby reducing the volume used and the direct cost of vaccine by 60–80 % compared with standard intramuscular vaccination (WHO 2010a). The method offers an equally safe and immunogenic alternative of vaccination at considerably reduced cost of a full course of PEP.

IDRV has been in use for several years in Thailand, Sri Lanka, and the Philippines. It has also been successfully introduced in India, where 13 states and union territories have already implemented it (WHO SEARO 2012).

5.4.1 Mechanism of Action of IDRV

IDRV involves deposition of approved rabies vaccine in the layers of dermis of skin. Subsequently the antigen is carried by antigen-presenting cells via the lymphatic drainage to the regional lymph nodes and later to the reticuloendothelial system eliciting a prompt and highly protective antibody response. Immunity is believed to depend mainly upon the CD4$^+$ T-cell-dependent neutralising antibody response to the G protein. In addition, cell-mediated immunity has long been reported as an important part of the defence against rabies. Cells presenting the fragments of G protein are the targets of cytotoxic T-cells and the N protein induced T-helper cells (NICD 2007). In IDRV, upon inoculating a small volume of vaccine (0.1 ml) at multiple sites, the antigen is directly presented to the antigen-presenting cells (without circulation/dilution in blood) at multiple sites triggering a stronger immune response. By intramuscular route, single dose consists of 0.5 ml or 1 ml of vaccine (depending upon the type) which is deposited in the muscles, and the antigen is then absorbed by the blood vessels and is presented to antigen-presenting cells which trigger immune response.

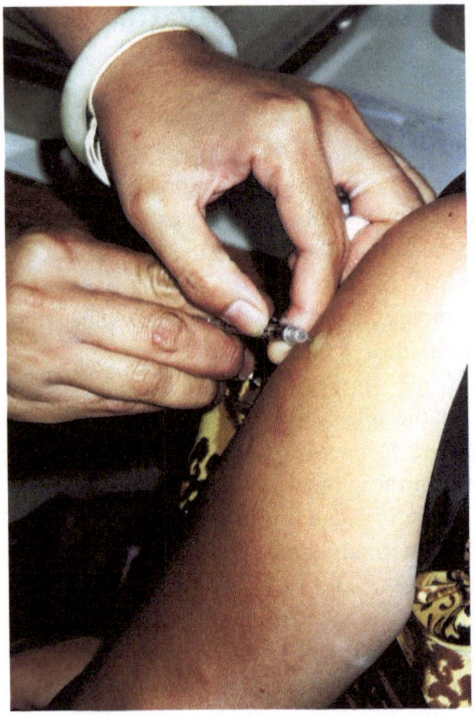

Fig. 5.4 Intradermal vaccination against rabies (Photo courtesy: Dr. Deborrah Briggs)

5.4.2 Intradermal Rabies Vaccines

Only the approved modern vaccines that meet the WHO requirements regarding safety, potency, and efficacy for this application may be used for IDRV. The vaccines for IDRV should meet the same WHO requirements for production and control as required for rabies vaccines delivered intramuscularly. In addition, the immunogenicity and safety of intradermally administered vaccines should be demonstrated in appropriate clinical trials using the WHO-recommended PEP regimen and a volume of 0.1 ml per intradermal site. To be approved for intradermal use, any new candidate vaccine should be proven potent (WHO 2010a, b). In India, the guidelines provide that the vaccine package leaflet should include a statement indicating that the potency as well as immunogenicity and safety allow safe use of the vaccine for pre-exposure and postexposure vaccination by intradermal route. Post-marketing surveillance data should be maintained for minimum of 2 years by the vaccine manufacturers on a predesigned and approved protocol (NICD 2007).

5.4.3 Intradermal Regimen for Rabies PEP

The WHO has recommended 2-site (2-2-2-0-2) intradermal PEP regimen for Category II and III exposures. The 2-site regimen prescribes injection of 0.1 ml intradermally at two different lymphatic drainage sites, usually the left and right upper arm, on days 0, 3, 7, and 28. The intradermal administration of vaccine must raise a visible and palpable 'bleb' in the skin (Fig. 5.4). In the event that a dose of vaccine is inadvertently given subcutaneously or intramuscularly, a new dose should be administered intradermally.

5.4.4 Vaccine Potency Requirements for Intradermal Route

The antigenic potency of all the vaccines which can be safely used by the intradermal route has proven similar and is well above the minimum value of 2.5 IU/ampoule. There is no evidence that intradermal administration requires vaccines with potency higher than that recommended for intramuscularly administered rabies vaccines. According to the WHO guidelines, the minimum potency requirement for human rabies vaccines for intradermal use should not be increased beyond 2.5 IU (per single intramuscular dose) by national authorities unless the need for a change is substantiated by clinical or field studies (WHO 2010a, b).

5.4.5 General Guidelines for IDRV

Intradermal vaccination is a skilled procedure. The following guidelines should be followed while carrying out the vaccination by intradermal route (NICD 2007; WHO 2010a):

- The vaccines should be an approved one for administration by intradermal route.
- Sufficient and adequately trained staff should be available to ensure correct storage and reconstitution of the vaccine and proper intradermal injection.
- Intradermal injections must be administered by staff trained in this technique.
- The reconstituted vaccine should be used as early as possible but within maximum 8 h.
- The vaccine should be stored at 2–8 °C and the unused vaccine must be discarded at the end of 6–8 h.
- Aseptic precautions should be followed while withdrawing the dose from the vial.
- The delivery of the vaccine should be proper. Vaccine when given intradermal should raise a visible and palpable bleb in the skin.
- In the event that the dose is inadvertently given subcutaneously or intramuscularly or in the event of spillage, a new dose should be given intradermal in nearby site.
- Rabies vaccines formulated with an adjuvant should not be administered intradermal.
- Animal bite victims on chloroquine therapy (antimalarial therapy) should be vaccinated by intramuscular route.

5.4.6 Material Requirement for Intradermal Vaccination

The following material is required for intradermal vaccination (NICD 2007):

- A vial of rabies vaccine approved for IDRV and its diluent
- A disposable 2 ml syringe with 24 G needle for reconstitution of vaccine
- Disposable 1 ml (insulin) syringe with graduations up to 100 or 40 units and with a fixed 28 G needle
- Disinfectant swabs (e.g. 70 % ethanol, isopropyl alcohol) for cleaning the top of the vial and the patient's skin

5.4.7 Intradermal Injection Technique

The freeze-dried vaccine in the vial is reconstituted aseptically with the diluent supplied by the manufacturer. With a 1 ml syringe, 0.2 ml of the vaccine is drawn for two intradermal injection sites at the rate of 0.1 ml for each site. The air bubbles are carefully expelled and it is ensured that there is no dead space in the syringe. For injecting the vaccine intradermally, the surface of the skin is stretched and the tip of the needle is inserted with bevel upwards, almost parallel to the skin surface. Half of the vaccine, i.e. 0.1 ml, is then slowly injected into the uppermost dermal layer of skin, over the deltoid area, preferably an inch above the insertion of the deltoid muscle. If the needle is correctly placed inside the dermis, considerable resistance is felt while injecting the vaccine. A raised papule should begin to appear immediately causing an orange peel appearance. The remaining half of the vaccine (0.1 ml) is injected on the opposite deltoid area. If the vaccine is injected too deeply into the skin (subcutaneous), a papule is not seen. In such case, the needle should be withdrawn and reinserted at an adjacent site and intradermal vaccine should be injected correctly again (NICD 2007).

5.4.8 Antirabies Treatment Centres for IDRV

Since it is to be ensured that the opened vial of vaccine should be used within 6–8 h, it is essential that individuals in sufficient numbers are available for vaccination at the vaccination centre to consume an opened vial fully. Otherwise the vaccine will be wasted and the very purpose of reducing the cost of vaccination will be defeated. For this reason, particular antirabies treatment centres have been specified in India to carry out intradermal vaccination. These centres are required to meet the following criteria (NICD 2007):

- They should have adequately trained staff for IDRV.
- They should be able to maintain cold chain for vaccine storage.
- They should have adequate supply of suitable syringes and needles for IDRV.
- They should be adequately trained in the management of open vials and safe storage practices.

5.5 Chemotherapy

Although rabies is preventable with PEP vaccination, there is no specific treatment for rabies infection after the onset of symptoms of the disease. When the disease is not treated, death typically occurs within 5–7 days after the symptoms appear. Medical management generally focusing on palliative care may prolong survival of the patient but even with advanced supportive care, the disease is usually always fatal.

A very small number of people have survived rabies till date. Prior to 2004, five people had been reported to survive after receiving immunoprophylaxis before the onset of symptoms (CDC 2005). However, in 2004, an adolescent female treated with a novel protocol in Wisconsin (USA) became the first person to survive documented clinical rabies without previous vaccination (Willoughby et al. 2005). The patient was a 15-year-old girl who was bitten by a bat on her left index finger while rescuing and releasing it. Clinical rabies developed 1 month after the incidence. The treatment included induction of coma while a native immune response matured; rabies vaccine was not administered. The patient was treated with ketamine, midazolam, ribavirin, and amantadine. Probable drug-related toxic effects included haemolysis, pancreatitis, acidosis, and hepatotoxicity. Lumbar puncture after 8 days showed an increased level of rabies antibody, and sedation was tapered. Paresis and sensory denervation then resolved. The patient was removed from isolation after 31 days and discharged to her home after 76 days. At nearly 5 months after her initial hospitalisation, she was alert and communicative but with choreoathetosis, dysarthria, and an unsteady gait (Willoughby et al. 2005).

This case represented the sixth known occurrence of human recovery after rabies infection till that time; however, the case was unique because the patient received no rabies prophylaxis either before or after the onset of illness. The five previous patients who survived were either previously vaccinated or received some form of PEP before the onset of illness (CDC 2005). This new therapeutic approach suggested that successful interventions may be possible; however, a number of patients subsequently treated in a similar way did not survive (van Thiel et al. 2009).

In 2009, another unvaccinated adolescent girl aged 17 years with a history of bat exposure 2 months before illness, symptoms of encephalitis, and positive rabies virus serology recovered from a presumed abortive rabies (defined as recovery from rabies without intensive care) after receiving only basic supportive care in Texas (CDC 2010a). Although the patient required multiple hospitalisations and follow-up visits for recurrent neurological symptoms, she survived without intensive care. Initially the patient was diagnosed as a case of suspected infectious encephalitis and was treated with intravenous acyclovir, ceftriaxone, ethambutol, isoniazid, pyrazinamide, and rifampin. However, efforts of the healthcare team for establishing the aetiology of encephalitis elicited the history of bat exposure. She recalled that about 2 months before her headaches began, she had entered a cave while on a camping trip in Texas and came into contact with flying bats. Although several bats hit her body, she did not notice any bites or scratches. Rabies was thus put in the differential diagnosis list.

The patient reportedly had never received rabies prophylaxis. Antibodies to rabies virus were detected in specimens of the girl's serum and cerebrospinal fluid (CSF) by indirect fluorescent antibody test (IFA), but the presence of rabies virus neutralisation antibodies (VNA) was not detected. Later, after notification of positive rabies serology results, the girl received one dose of rabies vaccine and 1,500 IU of HRIG. Additional doses of vaccine were not administered because of concern over possible adverse effects from potentiating the immune response. Later, the patient's serum tested positive for rabies VNA by RFFIT, whereas her CSF remained negative for rabies VNA.

The patient was managed supportively and never required intensive care. This is the first reported case in which certain clinical and serological findings indicate abortive human rabies. In all previous rabies survivors, the clinical courses were substantially longer, with more severe neurological compromise and more prominent stimulation of the immune system, including the induction of VNA. In this case, the clinical manifestation was relatively mild, which might imply variables associated with viral dose, route, and type, with a more limited virus replication and less apparent stimulation of the immune system (CDC 2010a).

Recently, another rabies patient entered the select list of survivors. An 8-year-old girl from rural California, who became infected with rabies after contact with free-roaming unvaccinated cats, is the third unvaccinated person to recover from clinical rabies in the USA (CDC 2012). The girl suffering from a sore throat, difficulty in swallowing, and weakness was ultimately diagnosed with rabies-based symptoms of paralysis, encephalitis, and a positive result on a test for rabies virus antibodies.

With a presumptive diagnosis of rabies, the patient was sedated with ketamine and midazolam and started on amantadine and nimodipine to prevent cerebral artery vasospasm, and fludrocortisone and hypertonic saline to maintain her sodium at a level >140 mmol/L. Neither HRIG nor rabies vaccine was administered. After the girl was put into an induced coma to prevent neurological complications of rabies infection until her body could clear the virus, and given other advanced supportive care, she recovered after 52 days in the hospital.

In this case, early diagnosis also might have affected the clinical outcome by focusing treatment at an early stage (CDC 2012). It has been recommended by the CDC that clinicians caring for patients with acute progressive encephalitis should consider rabies in the differential diagnosis and coordinate with health departments for laboratory diagnostic testing when indicated. Once a diagnosis of rabies has been established, clinical management should focus primarily on comfort care and adequate sedation of the patient (Jackson et al. 2003; CDC 2008). Experimental treatment might be considered after detailed discussions and informed consent by the patient, family, or legal representatives, particularly if the patient is young, healthy, and at an early stage of clinical disease (CDC 2008).

5.6 Postexposure Treatment Failures in Animal Bite Cases

PEP treatment is a proven method of rabies prevention. However, rabies-related deaths despite PEP administration are encountered. The treatment failures resulting in rabies are largely due to deviations from the guidelines laid down by the WHO. Delay in starting or failure to complete correct prophylaxis, particularly when the animal bites involve highly innervated regions, such as the head, neck, or hands, or following multiple wounds, may be the major reason of failure of prophylactic treatment (Wilde 2007; APCRI 2009; WHO 2010a). Some other reasons are listed in Box 5.1.

Box 5.1 Major Reasons for Treatment Failures Resulting in Human Rabies (APCRI 2009)

- Extensive deep bite cases with inoculation of rabies virus directly into the nerve, especially in bites on head, neck, and face (high-risk bites)
- Delay in starting treatment due to late reporting of patients
- Improper bite wound management
- Application of irritants to bite wounds
- Suturing of bite wounds without local infiltration of RIG
- Skipping RIG in cases where its administration is indicated
- Incomplete infiltration of wounds with RIG or missing some wounds
- Wrong administration of RIG (intramuscular injection instead of infiltration of wounds)
- Incomplete regimen of vaccination
- Failure to observe the vaccination schedule
- Administration of rabies vaccines into gluteal (hip) region instead of deltoid (arm) muscle
- Immunocompromised status of patient

Apart from failures due to omissions and flaws in PEP, rarely, true failures have also been reported despite administration of the state-of-the-art treatment (Shantavasinkul et al. 2010; WHO 2010a). Shantavasinkul et al. (2010) reported a case where the patient had rabies despite receiving appropriate treatment. The patient was bitten by a rabid dog on his hands and right knee. He received proper wound care, vaccination, and HRIG administration within 6 h after the attack. Although there were difficulties in infiltrating the wound at the nail bed of the right thumb, a great effort was made by experienced staff to infiltrate this wound with HRIG. The only deviation from the current WHO guidelines was the additional HRIG infiltration of the wounds 4 days after the first treatment when the positive results of the fluorescent antibody test of dog brain specimens became known. Nevertheless, the patient was able to mount a good antibody response, as his neutralising antibody level on day 27 was 1.39 IU/ml by RFFIT, which was much higher than 0.5 IU/ml, the level considered adequate for protection from rabies. The HRIG potency was reassessed and found to be comparable (280 IU/ml) with that of the manufacturer's export certificate (150–300 IU/ml). However, despite the treatment, the patient became symptomatic 24 days after being bitten.

This case raised the possibility of an unusual strain of rabies or other lyssavirus as cause of the disease. It also suggested that in canine rabies-endemic countries, physicians need to be aware of atypical presentations of human rabies (Shantavasinkul et al. 2010).

5.7 Management of Rabies Exposure in Animals

In animals, if the bite is seen, irrigation of the wound with 20 % soft soap solution or a solution of Zephiran immediately after exposure may prevent the establishment of the infection. No treatment should be attempted after clinical signs are evident (Radostits et al. 2007). Unlike humans, postexposure vaccination may not be of value in animals, as death usually occurs before appreciable immunity develops. Further, antirabies serum may not be available for animal treatment. The suspect animals should not be euthanised, particularly if human exposure has occurred; rather these should be isolated and kept under strict observation to note any sign of development of rabies. It will help to establish a diagnosis and take appropriate action for protection of the humans and animals that had previously come in contact with the affected animals (Radostits et al. 2007).

The National Association of State Public Health Veterinarians (NASPHV) publishes a Compendium of Animal Rabies Prevention and Control annually detailing the postexposure management of any animal exposed to a confirmed or suspected rabid animal (NASPHV 2011). Any animal potentially exposed to rabies virus by a wild, carnivorous mammal or bat that is not available for testing should be regarded as having been exposed to rabies. The Compendium provides guidance for management of dogs, cats, ferrets, and livestock that have been exposed to rabies. The suggested actions differ depending on the type of animal and the vaccination status at the time of exposure as shown below.

5.7.1 Dogs, Cats, and Ferrets

Any illness in an exposed animal should be reported immediately to the local health department. If signs suggestive of rabies develop (e.g. paralysis, seizures), the animal should be euthanised and the head sent for testing. The guidelines given by NASPHV (2011) for animals with different status of pre-exposure vaccination are summarised below.

Unvaccinated dogs, cats, and ferrets. Dogs, cats, and ferrets that have never been vaccinated and are exposed to a rabid animal should be euthanised immediately. If the owner is unwilling to have this done, the animal should be placed in strict isolation for 6 months. Isolation in this context refers to confinement in an enclosure that precludes direct contact with people and other animals. Rabies vaccine should be administered upon entry into isolation or up to 28 days before release to comply with pre-exposure vaccination recommendations. PEP of previously unvaccinated domestic animals is not practised in the USA as there is evidence that the use of vaccine alone will not reliably prevent the disease in these animals (Radostits et al. 2007; NASPHV 2011).

Dogs, cats, and ferrets overdue for booster vaccination. The animals which are overdue for a booster vaccination should be evaluated on a case-by-case basis considering the severity of exposure, time elapsed since last vaccination, number of previous vaccinations, current health status, and local rabies epidemiology to determine need for euthanasia or immediate revaccination and observation/isolation (NASPHV 2011).

Dogs, cats, and ferrets that are currently vaccinated. Dogs, cats, and ferrets that are currently vaccinated should be revaccinated immediately, kept under the owner's control, and observed for 45 days for development of any signs of rabies. This observation period is important to rule out any chances of vaccination failure due to any reasons and possibility of a vaccinated animal to contract rabies (NASPHV 2011). In case of progression of disease, rabies is most likely to become apparent within this period. The factors such as extensive exposure leading to overwhelming viral challenge, incomplete vaccine efficacy, improper vaccine administration, variable host immunocompetence, and immune-mediated fatality may result in reduction or loss of efficacy of the pre-exposure vaccination.

5.7.2 Livestock

All species of livestock are susceptible to rabies. Any illness in an exposed animal should be reported immediately to the concerned departments. If signs suggestive of rabies develop, the animal should be euthanised and the head dispatched for testing (NASPHV 2011).

Unvaccinated livestock. Unvaccinated livestock should be euthanised immediately. If the animal is not euthanised, it should be observed and confined on a case-by-case basis for 6 months.

Currently vaccinated livestock. Livestock exposed to a rabid animal and currently vaccinated with an approved vaccine for that species should be revaccinated immediately and observed for 45 days.

In contact animals in the herd. Multiple rabid animals in a herd or herbivore-to-herbivore transmission are uncommon; therefore, restricting the rest of the herd if a single animal has been exposed to or infected by rabies is usually not necessary.

5.7.3 Other Animals

Other mammals exposed to a rabid animal should be euthanised immediately. Animals maintained in licensed research facilities or accredited zoological parks should be evaluated on a case-by-case basis in consultation with public health authorities. Management options may include isolation, observation, or administration of rabies biologicals (NASPHV 2011).

References

Abazeed ME, Cinti S (2007) Rabies prophylaxis for pregnant women. Emerg Infect Dis 13:1966–1967

APCRI (2009) Manual on rabies immunoglobulin (RIG) administration, 1st edn. Association for Prevention and Control of Rabies in India, Bangalore

Bernard KW, Fishbein DB, Miller KD, Parker RA, Waterman S, Sumner JW, Reid FL, Johnson BK, Rollins AJ, Oster CN, Schonberger LB, Baer GM, Winkler WG (1985) Pre-exposure rabies immunization with human diploid cell vaccine: decreased antibody responses in persons immunized in developing countries. Am J Trop Med Hyg 34:633–647

Briggs DJ, Banzhoff A, Nicolay U, Sirikwin S, Dumavibhat B, Tongswas S, Wasi C (2000) Antibody response of patients after postexposure rabies vaccination with small intradermal doses of purified chick embryo cell vaccine or purified Vero cell rabies vaccine. Bull WHO 78:693–698

CDC (2005) Recovery of a patient from clinical rabies – Wisconsin, 2004. Morb Mortal Wkly Rep 53(50): 1171–1173

CDC (2008) Human rabies prevention – United States, 2008: recommendations of the advisory committee on immunization practices. Morb Mortal Wkly Rep 57(RR03):1–26, 28

CDC (2010a) Presumptive abortive human rabies-Texas, 2009. Morb Mortal Wkly Rep 59(7):185–190

CDC (2010b) Use of a reduced (4-dose) vaccine schedule for postexposure prophylaxis to prevent human rabies. Recommendations of the advisory committee on immunization practices. Morb Mortal Wkly Rep 59(RR02):1–9

CDC (2012) Recovery of a patient from clinical rabies – California, 2011. Morb Mortal Wkly Rep 61(4):64–65

CDCB (2012) Rabies: protocol for management of human rabies and management of animal exposures to prevent human rabies 2012. Communicable Disease Control Branch, Manitoba Government, Manitoba. http://www.gov.mb.ca/health/publichealth/cdc/protocol/rabies_protocol.pdf. Accessed 30 Aug 2012

Dobardzic A, Izurieta H, Woo EJ, Iskander J, Shadomy S, Rupprecht C, Ball R, Braun MM (2007) Safety review of the purified chick embryo cell rabies vaccine: Data from the Vaccine Adverse Event Reporting System (VAERS), 1997–2005. Vaccine 25:4244–4251

Dreesen DW, Bernard KW, Parker RA, Deutsch AJ, Brown J (1986) Immune complex-like disease in 23 persons following a booster dose of rabies human diploid cell vaccine. Vaccine 4:45–49

Fishbein DB, Dreesen DW, Holmes DF, Pacer RE, Ley AB, Yager PA, Sumner JW, Reid-Sanden FL, Sanderlin DW, Tong TC, Kemp DT (1989) Human diploid cell rabies vaccine purified by zonal centrifugation: A controlled study of antibody response and side-effects following primary and booster pre-exposure immunizations. Vaccine 7:437–442

Florida Department of Health (2012) Rabies prevention and control in Florida, 2012. Florida Department of Health, USA. http://www.doh.state.fl.us/environment/newsroom/brochures/rabiesguide2012.pdf. Accessed 30 Aug 2012

Georgia Department of Community Health (2011) Georgia rabies control manual, 6th edn. Georgia Department of Community Health, USA. http://health.state.ga.us/pdfs/epi/zvbd/Rabies%20Manual%202010_FINAL.pdf. Accessed 5 July 2012

Jackson AC, Warrell MJ, Rupprecht CE, Ertl HCJ, Dietzschold B, O'Reilly M, Leach RP, Fu ZF, Wunner WH, Bleck TP, Wilde H (2003) Management of rabies in humans. Clin Infect Dis 36:60–63

Lang J, Cetre JC, Picot N, Lanta M, Briantais P, Vital S, Le Mener V, Lutsch C, Rotivel Y (1998) Immunogenicity and safety in adults of a new chromatographically purified Vero-cell rabies vaccine (CPRV): a randomized, double-blind trial with purified Vero-cell rabies vaccine (PVRV). Biologicals 26:299–308

NASPHV (2011) Compendium of animal rabies prevention and control, 2011. National Association of State Public Health Veterinarians, recommendations and reports. Morb Mortal Wkly Rep 60(RR06):1–14

NICD (2007) National guidelines for rabies prophylaxis and intra-dermal administration of cell culture rabies vaccines. National Institute of Communicable Diseases, New Delhi

Pappaioanou M, Fishbein DB, Dreesen DW, Schwartz IK, Campbell GH, Sumner JW, Patchen LC, Brown WJ (1986) Antibody response to preexposure human diploid-cell rabies vaccine given concurrently with chloroquine. N Engl J Med 314:280–284

Partners for Rabies Prevention (2010) Blueprint for rabies prevention and control. http://www.rabiesblueprint.com/. Accessed 12 Apr 2012

Quiambao BP, Dimaano EM, Ambas C, Davis R, Banzhoff A, Malerczyk C (2005) Reducing the cost of post-exposure rabies prophylaxis: efficacy of 0.1 ml PCEC rabies vaccine administered intradermally using the Thai Red Cross post-exposure regimen in patients severely exposed to laboratory-confirmed rabid animals. Vaccine 23:1709–1714

Radostits OM, Gay CC, Hinchcliff KW, Constable PD (2007) Veterinary medicine – a textbook of the diseases of cattle, horses, sheep, pigs and goats, 10th edn. Saunders-Elsevier, Edinburgh

Rupprecht CE, Briggs D, Brown CM, Franka R, Katz SL, Kerr HD, Lett S, Levis R, Meltzer MI, Schaffner W, Cieslak PR (2009) Evidence for a 4-dose vaccine schedule for human rabies postexposure prophylaxis in previously non-vaccinated individuals. Vaccine 27:7141–7148

Shantavasinkul P, Tantawichien T, Wacharapluesadee S, Jeamanukoolkit A, Udomchaisakul P, Chattranukulchai P, Wongsaroj P, Khawplod P, Wilde H, Hemachudha T (2010) Failure of rabies postexposure prophylaxis in patients presenting with unusual manifestations. Clin Infect Dis 50:77–79

Sudarshan MK, Giri MS, Mahendra BJ, Venkatesh GM, Sanjay TV, Narayana DH, Ravish HS (2007) Assessing the safety of post-exposure rabies immunization in pregnancy. Hum Vaccine 3:87–89

Thisyakorn U, Pancharoen C, Ruxrungtham K, Ubolyam S, Khawplod P, Tantawichien T, Phanuphak P, Wilde H (2000) Safety and immunogenicity of pre-exposure rabies vaccination in children infected with human immunodeficiency virus type 1. Clin Infect Dis 30:218

van Thiel PP, de Bie RMA, Eftimov F, Tepaske R, Zaaijer HL, van Doornum GJJ, Schutten M, Osterhaus ADME, Majoie CBLM, Aronica E, Fehlner-Gardiner C, Wandeler AI, Kager PA (2009) Fatal human rabies due to Duvenhage virus from a bat in Kenya: failure of treatment with coma-induction, ketamine, and antiviral drugs. PLoS Negl Trop Dis 3(7):e428. doi:10.1371/journal.pntd.0000428

WHO (2005) WHO expert consultation on rabies. First report, WHO technical report series, no. 931. World Health Organization, Geneva

WHO (2010a) Rabies vaccines: WHO position paper. Wkly Epidemiol Rec No 32 85:309–320

WHO (2010b) WHO guide for rabies pre and post-exposure prophylaxis in humans (revised 15 June 2010). Department of Neglected Tropical Diseases, World Health Organization, Geneva

WHO (2011) The immunological basis for immunization series. Module 17: rabies. Immunization, vaccines and biologicals. World Health Organization, Geneva

WHO (2012) Current strategies for human rabies pre and post-exposure prophylaxis. Guide for post-exposure prophylaxis (PEP). http://www.who.int/rabies/human/WHO_strategy_prepost_exposure/en/index1.html. Accessed 15 Aug 2012

WHO SEARO (2012) Rabies: Country profile: India. World Health Organization, Regional Office for South-East Asia, New Delhi. http://www.searo.who.int/LinkFiles/Zoonoses_IND-rabies-cp.pdf. Accessed 15 Aug 2012

Wilde H (2007) Failures of rabies post-exposure prophylaxis. Vaccine 25:7605–7609

Willoughby RE Jr, Tieves KS, Hoffman GM, Ghanayem NS, Amelie-Lefond CM, Schwabe MJ, Chusid MJ, Rupprecht CE (2005) Survival after treatment of rabies with induction of coma. N Engl J Med 352:2508–2514

6 Vaccines and Other Biologicals

Abstract

Louise Pasteur prepared the first crude nerve tissue vaccine for rabies. Dr. David Semple developed the completely inactivated and safer Semple vaccine at Central Research Institute in Kasauli (India). With the advent of modern cell culture vaccines, the WHO does not advocate the use of the earlier nerve tissue vaccines anymore. Modern vaccines produced on various cellular substrates and continuous cell lines are highly effective in both pre-exposure and postexposure prophylaxis against rabies. Different novel vaccines such as attenuated rabies mutants, viral recombinant vaccines, DNA vaccines, and subunit vaccines have been developed recently that hold great promise for the future. The use of rabies immunoglobulin (RIG) for passive immunisation also dates back to the nineteenth century. Currently two types of products, namely, equine RIG and human RIG, are available. Development of alternative products and MAb is underway. There has also been considerable progress in the production of rabies vaccines for animal use. Several types of vaccines are available for administration to domestic animals or wild species by parenteral or oral routes. A third generation of live veterinary rabies vaccine has been developed more recently using recombinant technology.

6.1 Human Vaccines and Other Biologicals

Louis Pasteur developed the earliest effective vaccine against rabies. He and his colleagues traced infected brain and spinal cord as a major replicative source of the causative agent of rabies. They were able to fix the causative agent by serial passage in rabbits through intracranial inoculation. After a series of experiments, the first course of successful rabies prophylaxis was administered by Pasteur to a boy, Joseph Meister, in the year 1885 (Wu et al. 2011b). The method involved inoculation with homogenates of the rabies virus-infected rabbit spinal cord that had been progressively desiccated in sterile air. The recipient initially received a subcutaneous injection of the homogenate that was fully inactivated. This was followed by a series of injections of preparations that contained progressively more virulent virus (Wu et al. 2011b; Hicks et al. 2012). This led to the development of nerve tissue vaccines. Pasteur's method was used for more than half a century, before significant modifications were

S.R. Garg, *Rabies in Man and Animals*, DOI 10.1007/978-81-322-1605-6_6,

introduced in rabies vaccine preparation (Wu et al. 2011b). The developments in the rabies vaccine production have been comprehensively reviewed by Nandi and Kumar (2010), Wu et al. (2011b), and Hicks et al. (2012).

6.1.1 Old Vaccines

6.1.1.1 Nerve Tissue Vaccines

The first crude nerve tissue vaccine for rabies was prepared by Pasteur. The vaccine was not consistently inactivated and comprised of a mixture of inactivated and live virus, which led in some cases to recipients developing rabies possibly from the vaccination virus (Wu et al. 2011b; Hicks et al. 2012). Moreover, it was difficult to produce sufficient vaccine from rabbits to meet the requirement. That led to the development of the Fermi vaccine and Semple vaccine in sheep and goats. Fermi and Semple used phenol to inactivate the rabies virus in nerve tissue. Fermi vaccine was a 5 % aqueous suspension of rabies virus-infected sheep or goat brain, treated with 0.5–1 % phenol at 22 °C, but was still a combination of live and inactivated virus. Dr. David Semple, who observed that Fermi vaccine was totally inactivated by phenol at 30 °C for 48–72 h (Semple 1911), developed completely inactivated vaccine in the year 1911 at Central Research Institute, Kasauli in India, which was a major historical improvement in the rabies vaccine safety. Semple vaccine contained 5–10 % of sheep or goat brain tissue, 0.25–0.5 % phenol, and possibly 1:10,000 thiomersal as preservative (Wu et al. 2011b).

All these vaccines were prepared in the adult mammal nervous tissue. Myelin present in these caused sensitisation and encephalitis in the patients. Observing that the substances responsible for side effects were largely absent in the newborn animal tissue, suckling mouse brain vaccine was subsequently developed to minimise the adverse reactions of the nerve tissue vaccine. Fuenzalida et al. (1964) introduced an inactivated rabies vaccine prepared as a 1 % homogenised neonatal mouse brain suspension (Fuenzalida et al. 1964). Though an improvement over the adult nerve tissue vaccines, severe adverse reactions were reported with this vaccine too (Bonito et al. 2004).

The World Health Organization (WHO) does not advocate the use of nerve tissue vaccines, so the production of Semple vaccine has been completely stopped in India, but it is still produced and used in some Asian and African countries. Suckling mouse brain vaccine is also in use in some Latin American countries (Wu et al. 2011b).

6.1.1.2 Avian Embryo-Derived Vaccines

Chicken embryo-derived rabies vaccines were evolved to overcome the problem of reactogenic nature of nerve tissue vaccines. The rabies virus Flury strain was adapted to 1-day-old chicks and subsequently established in chick embryos and passaged in embryonated chicken egg (Leach and Johnson 1940; Koprowski and Cox 1948; Wu et al. 2011b). The Flury low egg passage (LEP) vaccine consisted of live virus at the 40–50th egg passage level and was lyophilised from a 33 % whole-embryo suspension. The LEP vaccine was used in mass dog vaccination campaigns but retained residual virulence and occasionally caused rabies in young puppies, cats, and cattle. The Flury high egg passage (HEP, 180th passage or above) vaccine was tested in humans during the 1950s and 1960s but was eventually discontinued due to unreliable potency and a sense of 'little practical importance' (Fox et al. 1957; Wu et al. 2011b).

A duck embryo-derived rabies vaccine was developed in the 1950s (Peck et al. 1955; Wu et al. 2011b). This vaccine was a rather crude 10 % suspension of whole embryos, inactivated using β-propiolactone. It was used extensively in humans in the USA for about 25 years, until the early 1980s. However, even this vaccine was not entirely successful as significant poor antigenic responses and severe adverse reactions were associated with it (Vodopija and Clarke 1991; Wu et al. 2011b).

6.1.2 New-Generation Modern Vaccines

The old method of vaccination for protection against rabies involved administration of the rabies virus antigens in homogenised tissue suspensions. These unpurified nerve tissue or whole avian embryo vaccines do not meet the modern quality standards, and their administration to humans may be regarded as an unacceptable practice (Wu et al. 2011b).

The development of cell culture for virus propagation dramatically changed the scenario of vaccination against rabies. The first tissue culture rabies vaccine for use in humans was derived from virus grown in primary hamster kidney cells; however, its application was limited (Wu et al. 2011b). During the late 1970s and the 1980s, different types of vaccines were prepared on various cellular substrates such as primary explant cells of hamster, dog, or foetal calf kidney; fibroblasts of chicken embryo; diploid cells from rhesus monkey foetal lung; human diploid cells; and finally cells from continuous lines (Vero cells).

The production of some of these vaccines was stopped at the end of the 1980s while others continued. Since their development more than four decades ago, concentrated and purified cell culture and embryonated egg-based rabies vaccines have proven to be safe and effective in preventing rabies. Intended for use both for pre-exposure prophylaxis and for postexposure prophylaxis (PEP), these vaccines have been administered to millions of people worldwide (WHO 2012).

The historical perspective of development of modern cell culture vaccines has been elaborately reviewed by Wu et al. (2011b). A brief account of the most common rabies vaccines traded internationally today is given below.

6.1.2.1 Human Diploid Cell Vaccine (HDCV)

An inactivated rabies vaccine for human use was first prepared in cell culture in 1964. In 1966 it was shown that the human diploid cell strain WI-38 was a suitable substrate for the propagation of the Pitman-Moore strain of fixed rabies virus. Later, its production was done in MRC-5 cell line, a similar but foetal lung cell strain developed in Europe. The vaccine was first licensed for use in France in 1974 and commercial production started in 1978. In the USA, the vaccine was licensed in 1980. HDCV was the first purified, concentrated, and lyophilised rabies vaccine without any adjuvant, but containing human serum albumin as a stabiliser. Thereafter, rabies HDCV was recommended as a gold standard reference vaccine by the WHO. Compared to other rabies vaccines, HDCV caused much fewer adverse effects (Wu et al. 2011b; WHO 2012). However, despite the safety and high immunogenicity of these vaccines, the relatively low titre of virus production by human diploid cells posed a problem in large-scale production of a comparatively cheap rabies vaccine of equal quality. Therefore, the cost of HDCV remains high, and its availability is limited typically to developed countries (Wu et al. 2011b; WHO 2012).

A concentrated rabies vaccine adsorbed (RVA) was developed in FRhL-2 cells, i.e. foetal rhesus monkey lung cells in 1982, and used in the USA. Although licensed, RVA is no longer available on the US market. Interestingly, the vaccine was redeveloped and licensed for human use in 2002 in India (Wu et al. 2011b). It is presently manufactured and marketed by the Serum Institute of India under the brand name Rabivax.

6.1.2.2 Purified Vero Cell Rabies Vaccine (PVRV)

A Vero cell line was established in 1962 from African green monkey kidney cells. Following the production of the inactivated poliomyelitis vaccine in Vero cells, studies were carried out to develop a human rabies vaccine. Rabies vaccine cultured in Vero cells was developed in the early 1980s. The vaccine, which required a purification step in order to remove the residual cellular DNA, is known as the purified Vero cell rabies vaccines (PVRV). PVRV was licensed in Europe in 1985. Currently, PVRV is widely available and commonly used worldwide, including India, but is not licensed for use in the USA (Wu et al. 2011b; WHO 2012).

6.1.2.3 Purified Chick Embryo Cell Vaccine (PCECV)

This vaccine is prepared in primary chick embryo cells derived from specific pathogen-free eggs. It is a freeze-dried preparation consisting of purified and concentrated rabies virus antigen inactivated with β-propiolactone (WHO 2012). PCECV was developed initially using Flury HEP virus in 1972. Another PCECV was developed using the Flury LEP virus. After more than a decade of inactivated LEP vaccine application in dogs, the seed virus was further adapted to chicken embryo fibroblast cells and then developed into the second PCECV for humans. Currently, PCECV is one of the most commonly used human rabies vaccines (Wu et al. 2011b).

6.1.2.4 Purified Duck Embryo Vaccine (PDEV)

Owing to the need for improvements in the whole duck embryo-derived tissue vaccine, purified duck embryo vaccine (PDEV) was developed. The vaccine is registered in some European and Asian countries, but not licensed in the USA (Wu et al. 2011b). The vaccine was introduced in India to meet the ever increasing need for modern rabies vaccines. Though PDEV is in strict sense not a cell culture vaccine (infected duck embryos are homogenised and viruses are purified by zonal centrifugation and inactivated with β-propiolactone), it is considered on par with any cell culture vaccine by the WHO. PDEV was originally manufactured by Berna Biotech, Switzerland, under the brand name of Lyssavac N. Following the transfer of technology in 2001, the same PDEV is now being manufactured in India by the Zydus Cadila Ltd., marketed as Vaxirab from 2003 onwards. The vaccine has been approved by the Drug Controller General of India. PDEV manufactured in India is being exported to some Asian countries under the brand name of Lyssavac N. Studies in India have concluded that indigenously manufactured PDEV is a safe and immunogenic vaccine and can be safely used for PEP (Mahendra et al. 2010).

In India, currently, several private and public firms are producing and/or marketing modern antirabies vaccines. The features of some vaccines available in the country are given in Table 6.1.

6.1.3 Development of Newer Vaccines

Traditionally, rabies vaccines have been produced by serial passage of rabies virus in nerve tissue or cell culture until attenuated (live virus) or by inactivation of the virus (killed virus). Currently available new-generation vaccines against rabies are quite successful, but there have been numerous attempts to develop even better vaccines with greater features such as enhanced immunogenicity, rapid immune response, sustained protection with fewer (preferably single) prophylactic doses, lower cost of production, feasibility of large-scale commercial production, reasonable stability at room temperature, and reduced or no requirement of rabies immunoglobulin (RIG) application.

With the advancement in the molecular and genetic manipulation techniques, different novel vaccines for rabies have been developed recently that hold great promise for the future (Ertl 2009). Some of these are briefly described below.

6.1.3.1 Attenuated Rabies Mutants

Advancements in reverse genetics have facilitated production of reconstituted rabies viruses with altered genomes through expression of mutated genes. A number of attenuated rabies viruses have been generated and tested using such techniques (Ertl 2009). Wu et al. (2011a) recently described the development of a highly attenuated rabies virus ERAg3m, with a mutation in the glycoprotein (G) gene and a switch of the G gene with the matrix protein gene in the viral genome. After a one-dose intramuscular vaccination, the ERAg3m virus protected 100 % of mice and hamsters from lethal challenge (Wu et al. 2011a). It was shown that the live attenuated rabies virus when given pre-exposure or coinfected with street rabies virus was capable of preventing rabies in two different animal models. Overall, it offered better protection than the inactivated vaccine (Wu et al. 2011a).

Attenuated rabies mutants, in which crucial genes are deleted and replaced with a second glycoprotein gene, have been shown preclinically to induce more potent immune responses than

Table 6.1 Some human antirabies vaccines available in India

Brand name, manufacturer, product detail	Use, dosage, site, route of administration, packing detail[a]
Abhayrab (Human Biologicals Institute – a division of Indian Immunologicals Ltd.)	Use: pre-exposure and postexposure vaccination against rabies
Purified inactivated rabies vaccine, prepared on Vero cells, using L. Pasteur 2061/Vero rabies strain, freeze-dried vaccine	Pre-exposure prophylaxis: three immunising doses on 0, 7, and 21 or 28 days followed by annual booster
	Postexposure prophylaxis: one immunising dose on postexposure days 0, 3, 7, 14, 28, and 90 each
	Route: deep intramuscular route in the deltoid region or by subcutaneous route
	Packing: box of one-dose vial along with diluent ampoule (0.5 ml), sterile disposable syringe with needle, and vaccination card
Rabipur (Chiron Behring Vaccines Pvt. Ltd. – a Novartis company; marketed by Novartis)	Use: pre-exposure and postexposure vaccination against rabies
PCEC (purified chick embryo cell culture) rabies vaccine; the strain used for manufacture is Flury LEP strain of rabies virus, lyophilised	Dose and route: used as either intramuscular or intradermal and by all regimens permitted by the authorities in India for pre-exposure and postexposure prophylaxis
	Packing: 1 vial with lyophilised powder+1 ampoule with 1 ml sterile water for injection and 1 sterile disposable syringe and needle
SII Rabivax (Serum Institute of India Ltd.)	Use: pre-exposure and postexposure vaccination against rabies
Rabies vaccine (adsorbed), human diploid cell culture vaccine, liquid vaccine	Dosage:
Rabies virus (Pitman-Moore strain) adapted, grown on human diploid cells, and inactivated with β propiolactone; after inactivation the virus is adsorbed onto aluminium phosphate	Pre-exposure: one injection each on days 0, 7, 21, or 28; booster injection 1 year later and then every 5 years
	Postexposure: one injection each on day 0, 3, 7, 14, 28 each (total 5 injections)
	In those previously immunised: one injection each on day 0 and day 3
	Site: deltoid muscle or anterolateral aspect of the thigh in children
	Route of administration: IM use only
	Packing: one vial (1 ml, single dose) along with syringe and needle
Verorab (Sanofi Pasteur, France; marketed by Zuventus Healthcare Ltd., Mumbai)	Use: pre-exposure and postexposure vaccination against rabies
Inactivated purified Vero cell rabies vaccine, lyophilised, produced on Vero cells using rabies virus (Wistar Rabies PM/W138 1503-3 M strain)	Pre-exposure prophylaxis by intramuscular route: one dose each on days 0, 7, and 28 (or 21) followed by a booster injection after 1 year and then a booster every 5 years
	Postexposure prophylaxis by intramuscular route: one dose each on postexposure days 0, 3, 7, 14, and 28
	Postexposure prophylaxis by intradermal vaccination: one intradermal dose comprising of 0.1 ml of reconstituted vaccine (1/5 of the intramuscular dose) according to the approved regimen in India, i.e. the 2-site intradermal regimen (Thai Red Cross intradermal regimen, 2-2-2-0-2 regimen) that prescribes 1 injection of 0.1 ml each at 2 sites on days 0, 3, 7, and 28
	Packing: one dose in a vial+0.5 ml solvent in ampoule or prefilled syringe

[a]Based on the company's product information. Consult product literature, guidelines, and local regulations before use

traditional vaccines and the responses came up more rapidly. The virus while retaining full immunogenicity can be made completely non-pathogenic by deleting certain crucial genes, thus, obliterating the need of its inactivation. Such viral mutants may be highly suited to replace the current vaccines for PEP (Ertl 2009).

6.1.3.2 Viral Recombinant Vaccines

Cloning the rabies virus glycoprotein into bacterial plasmids through genetic manipulation and then expressing the protein in a range of systems provides an alternative potential approach for developing new vaccines against rabies (Hicks et al. 2012). The recombinant proteins expressed in a range of vectors in several studies have been shown to be protective in mouse models of vaccination and virus challenge. Viral vectors have also been explored as vaccine carriers; however, these have a limitation that the existing neutralising antibodies to the parental virus in the target species can inhibit the uptake of recombinant viral vectors and hence production of the vaccine antigen (Ertl 2009).

6.1.3.3 DNA Vaccines

DNA vaccines are bacterial plasmids constructed to express an encoded protein following in vivo administration and subsequent transfection of cells. The use of DNA vaccination in rabies prophylaxis has been demonstrated in a number of animal models since 1994, but the poor immunogenicity and requirement of higher DNA doses in larger animals limit its application. However, the progress and accomplishments in the field of vector design hold considerable promise for rabies DNA vaccine development (Ullas et al. 2012).

6.1.3.4 Subunit Vaccines

Glycoprotein is the major surface protein of rabies virus, responsible for the production of neutralising antibodies; hence the rabies virus glycoprotein has been the major target for subunit vaccine development to provide complete protection against rabies virus. The rabies virus glycoprotein has been expressed in various expression systems. Various recombinant protein expression platforms offer the advantage of obtaining scalable protein production without the necessity of handling live rabies virus (Ramya et al. 2011).

6.1.3.5 Replication-Deficient or Single-Cycle Live Rabies Virus-Based Vectors

Though live rabies virus vaccines have the greatest potential to induce strong immunity against rabies virus, their use poses risk of adverse effects of residual pathogenesis. The reverse genetics technologies have been used to develop replication-deficient or single-cycle live rabies virus-based vectors for use as a single-dose rabies vaccine for humans (McGettigan 2010). These vaccines have been shown to be efficacious and safe in animal models; however, additional studies are required before these could replace the current inactivated human rabies vaccines.

6.1.4 Potency and Safety of Modern Rabies Vaccines

The WHO published the requirements for rabies vaccine for human use in 1981 (WHO 1981). Later, an additional document 'WHO requirements for rabies vaccine (inactivated) for human use produced in continuous cell lines' was published in 1987 (WHO 1987). The former encompassed the requirements for vaccines derived from mammalian neural tissue as well as the vaccines produced using embryonated eggs and variety of cell substrates, whereas the latter covered only the vaccines produced in continuous cell lines. Subsequently in 1994, amendments which updated the section on the International Standards for Rabies Vaccine were published (WHO 1994a, b).

Keeping in view the subsequent developments in the production and quality control of vaccines as well as in their overall regulation, particularly the safety issues, the revision of the requirements for rabies vaccines was envisaged at the meetings of a working group held at WHO, Geneva, in May 2003 and May 2004 and the revised recommendations for inactivated rabies vaccine for human use produced in cell substrates and embryonated eggs were published (WHO 2007), replacing all previous requirements. The scope of these recommendations encompasses vaccines produced in cell substrates, ranging from primary cells (hamster kidney and chick embryo fibroblasts) and diploid cells to continuous cell lines such as Vero cells. Purified vaccines produced using duck embryos are also within the scope of the document. This document focuses on the recommendations for production, control, and evaluation of rabies vaccines. However, vaccines produced in mammalian neural tissues are not considered because their use is no longer recommended.

Besides the use of advanced techniques, the production of modern vaccines is also guided by the governing regulations and the basic criteria of efficacy, purity, potency, and safety. In the cell culture vaccine production, rabies virus is propagated in cell cultures, and the viral harvest is concentrated, purified, inactivated, and lyophilised. Inactivation of the vaccines is usually done with β-propiolactone, and the vaccines undergo the safety, sterility, potency, and stability tests. All cell culture vaccines need to have WHO-recommended minimum potency of 2.5 IU or more per single intramuscular dose. The shelf life of these vaccines is ≥3 years, provided they are stored at +2 °C to +8 °C and protected from sunlight (WHO 2010; Wu et al. 2011b).

The modern vaccines are highly effective in both pre-exposure and postexposure prophylaxis against rabies. The vaccines induce a prompt response to attain the WHO's specified minimum rabies virus-neutralising antibody titre of 0.5 IU/ml of serum. In healthy vaccinees, this level should be achieved in most individuals by day 14 of a postexposure regimen, with or without simultaneous administration of RIG and irrespective of age. The modern vaccines have good immunological memory (WHO 2010).

As the purity, potency, and safety of vaccines have increased over time, the number and frequency of doses required for successful prophylaxis have decreased. As against the nerve tissue vaccine which required daily doses over a 10- or 14-day period, the cell culture vaccines have only a five-dose regimen (Wu et al. 2011b).

6.1.5 Rabies Immunoglobulin (RIG)

Apart from active immunisation with vaccine, passive immunisation is also required in most instances in a rabies-infected area for the success of PEP. The use of RIG for passive immunisation dates back to 1890 when Babes demonstrated its utility in experimental animals. In 1945, Habel and his colleagues conclusively demonstrated that postexposure treatment with antirabies serum given at the site of the bite soon after virus injection, along with vaccine, was much more effective than the vaccine alone. Following similar reports, the WHO coordinated a series of experiments to determine the optimal dose of RIG, so that active immunity induced by vaccination is not significantly suppressed. The combined use of vaccine and serum became a standard postexposure treatment after the recommendation by the WHO in 1966 (APCRI 2009).

For production of RIG, several types of animals were used, but horses proved to be more suitable because large quantities could be obtained. Till 1960, equine rabies immunoglobulin (ERIG) in use was not purified and led to the incidence of serious side effects like anaphylaxis and serum sickness. In the late 1960s, highly purified and enzyme-digested ERIG became available. This has resulted in fewer side effects. While the production of human RIG (HRIG) was initiated by Hosty as early as in 1959, Cabasso standardised its production and determined the optimal dosage in 1971 (APCRI 2009).

Currently two types of products, namely, HRIG and ERIG, are available for passive immunisation, but the availability and access to HRIG is usually limited due to high cost, particularly in the developing countries. However, ERIG is quite a safe alternative option for use in the resource-poor countries. The currently available ERIG is a highly purified product and much safer than the previous generation heterologous products (WHO 2012).

6.1.5.1 Equine Rabies Immunoglobulin (ERIG)

Different types of ERIG have been produced using various immunogenic preparations, consisting usually of a combination of inactivated

Table 6.2 Some rabies immunoglobulins available in India

Brand name, manufacturer, product detail	Use, dosage, site, route of administration, packing detail[a]
Abhay RIG (Human Biologicals Institute – a division of Indian Immunologicals Ltd.)	Use: for passive immunisation against rabies (in conjunction with rabies vaccine)
Equine antirabies immunoglobulin fragments	Dose: 40 IU/Kg bodyweight. If anatomically feasible, as much as possible of the dose should be infiltrated around the wounds
	Route: intramuscular
	Packing: vials of 5 ml, each vial containing not less than 1,500 IU of equine antirabies immunoglobulin fragments
Equirab (Bharat Serums and Vaccines Ltd.)	Use: for passive immunisation against rabies (in conjunction with rabies vaccine)
Rabies antiserum – equine antirabies immunoglobulin fragments	Dose: 40 IU/Kg bodyweight. If anatomically feasible, as much as possible of the dose should be infiltrated around the wounds
	Route: intramuscular
	Packing: vials of 5 ml, each vial containing not less than 1,000 IU of equine antirabies immunoglobulin fragments

[a]Based on the company's product information. Consult product literature, guidelines, and local regulations before use

and fixed strains of rabies virus. ERIG production involves immunising horses with immunogenic preparations, allowing adequate immunisation period and subsequent bleeding for collection of serum. Purification techniques are used to maximise the specific activity and to minimise the allergenic substances in the product with an objective to reduce the risk of sensitisation to heterologous ERIG. The availability of purified ERIG has reduced the incidence of serum sickness among the recipients (WHO 2012). In India, ERIG is indigenously produced from hyperimmunised horses both in the government sector and in the private sector.

Many of these preparations are now based on ERIG F(ab')2 fragments which constitute a specific part of the immunoglobulin that neutralises rabies virus. It is free from the reactogenic Fc fragment causing significant reduction in the occurrence of adverse reactions (APCRI 2009). Efficient separation of F(ab')2 fragments from Fc fragments and other serum proteins has been a challenge for industrial scale production despite the availability of several purification techniques. Some novel methods have been recently proposed to produce ERIG F(ab')(2) fragments from crude equine plasma (Fernandes et al. 2008; Kittipongwarakarn et al. 2011).

6.1.5.2 Human Rabies Immunoglobulin (HRIG)

HRIG preparations have been developed and used for postexposure treatment in most industrialised countries to avoid the reactions associated with ERIG. HRIG is homologous in origin and its infiltration does not require prior skin testing. Since 1975, this product has been administered to more than 250,000 people in the USA, and no cases of serum sickness have been reported (WHO 2012). HRIG has a longer half-life in comparison to ERIG, so its dose is half the dose of ERIG. As HRIG has slower clearance than F(ab')2 fragments from the body, it is advisable to use HRIG in multiple/severe exposures (APCRI 2009). However, HRIG is expensive, therefore, not as commonly available. In India, HRIG is imported and less accessible.

Recently, production of a functional humanised Fab fragment of a neutralising antibody against rabies virus has been described as a prototype of a therapeutic agent that could be an alternative to ERIG and HRIG obtained from the blood of vaccinated human donors (Sveshnikov et al. 2010).

Some RIG products available in India are mentioned in Table 6.2.

6.1.6 Development of Monoclonal Antibodies (MAb)

Limited supply of HRIG and ERIG is a major obstruction in the passive immunisation component of the PEP against rabies in the countries where canine rabies is endemic. Based on vaccine utilisation, it is estimated that in India alone about five million people receive PEP against rabies annually (WHO SEARO 2012). Replacement of HRIG and ERIG with other potentially cheaper and efficacious biologicals, therefore, remains a high priority. Development of alternative products and use of carefully selected MAb for therapeutic purpose provides a possible solution to the problem. MAb have demonstrated their activity in certain animal models and with the progress of technology, their potential ease of production in large quantities at low cost and ease of quality control compared to polyclonal serum make it an attractive proposition (Muller et al. 2009; WHO 2012).

The scientist of Crucell, a global biopharmaceutical company, Thomas Jefferson University (TJU) in Philadelphia, and the CDC collaborated to discover a combination of human MAb for the postexposure treatment of rabies (Anonymous 2012). The candidate MAb product is designed to be used together with rabies vaccine. Preclinical studies conducted during 2004 indicated that the MAb combination could neutralise (inactivate) rabies virus at least as effectively as HRIG. Since then, the rabies MAb combination has successfully progressed through phase I clinical trials in the USA and India (in 2006–2007) and phase II trials in the USA and the Philippines. An additional phase II study in India is now imminent. This study is designed to collect safety and neutralising activity data of the CL184 antibody in combination with the vaccine in simulated rabies PEP setting. Crucell and Sanofi Pasteur are codeveloping the rabies antibody product which is not derived from blood and would be affordable for everyone. Other important potential advantages of this MAb product compared to RIG include more consistent production volumes and less painful administration due to smaller injections.

In yet another initiative, MassBiologics and the Serum Institute of India partnered in an effort to develop MAb that could be used in place of HRIG. The new cost-effective rabies therapy developed by them gave positive results from a phase 1 study carried out in India in the year 2010 (Anonymous 2010). The study showed that a new MAb (RAB-1) resulted in protective antibody levels in the serum of treated subjects. Preclinical testing of RAB-1 showed that it neutralised all isolates available from a panel of rabies viruses. In the phase 1 trial run at the King Edward Memorial (KEM) Hospital in Mumbai, 74 healthy volunteers were randomised into several groups that either received escalating doses of RAB-1 or of HRIG combined with vaccine. RAB-1 was well tolerated by all subjects, with no serious adverse side effects. Blood samples were then analysed and showed that the volunteers who received RAB-1 and vaccine at a dose of 0.150 mg/kg had levels of rabies antibodies equal to or higher than the levels from those volunteers who had received the standard dose of HRIG and vaccine. The half-life of RAB-1 was 18–19 days (Anonymous 2010). Blood samples were also analysed by the Kansas State Veterinary Diagnostic Laboratory to determine if antibodies present in the volunteers' bloodstream could neutralise rabies virus in a cell-based assay using two different strains of virus. The data showed that volunteers who received RAB-1 at 0.150 mg/kg with vaccine had similar or better protective serum levels when compared to those who received HRIG with vaccine.

Following the successful conclusion of this phase 1 trial, the Serum Institute of India and MassBiologics are moving ahead in a clinical trial in India to evaluate the efficacy of RAB-1 combined with vaccine compared to the standard of care for patients who have been exposed to potentially rabid animals. It will be possible to produce MAb in large quantities and at much lower costs than blood products, which could make this new therapy widely available in Asia and India (Anonymous 2010).

6.2 Animal Vaccines

There has been considerable progress during the past two decades in the production of rabies vaccines, whether live or inactivated, for animal use. With the increasing use of continuous cell lines as a substrate and adoption of the fermentor technology for antigen production, several types of second-generation vaccines are currently available for administration to domestic animals or wild species by parenteral or oral routes according to vaccine characteristics (WHO 2012). Highly immunogenic inactivated but affordable cell culture vaccines are widely available for immunisation of dogs via parenteral route, and more and more developing countries are coming forward for transfer or acquisition of modern cell culture technology for parenteral veterinary vaccine production.

More recently a third generation of live veterinary rabies vaccine has been developed using recombinant technology. Depending upon the expression system, these vaccines are used either parenterally or orally. Oral rabies vaccines are widely used in foxes in Europe and in raccoons in the USA. Trials are underway for oral immunisation of dogs in developing countries (WHO 2012).

6.2.1 Vaccines for Parenteral Use

Modified live-virus and inactivated vaccines are produced in cell culture, using either primary cells or continuous cell lines. The seed virus and cell systems may vary considerably between different manufacturers. Combined vaccines are already used for the immunisation of dogs and cats (WHO 2012). Several different antigens are incorporated in canine rabies vaccine, such as canine distemper, canine hepatitis, leptospirosis, and canine parvovirus. Combined rabies vaccines for cats may include various other antigens such as feline panleukopenia virus, feline calicivirus, and feline parvoviruses. A combined rabies and foot-and-mouth disease vaccine is available for use in cattle, sheep, and goats. Some commonly available animal rabies vaccines in India are listed in Table 6.3.

6.2.1.1 Potency Requirements

The eighth report of the WHO Expert Committee on Rabies in 1992 suggested that inactivated veterinary vaccines with a potency of less than 1.0 IU per dose, as measured by the NIH (National Institutes of Health) test, should not be licensed or released unless an adequately designed experiment has demonstrated a duration of immunity of at least 1 year in the species for which the vaccine is to be used. The potency of live and inactivated vaccines should be ascertained at intervals after they have been distributed. Inactivated vaccine, even in liquid form, and lyophilised modified live-virus vaccines are relatively stable when stored under proper conditions. It is recommended that samples from the field that are approaching their expiry date be tested to verify that storage conditions are adequate (WHO 2012).

6.2.2 Modified Live-Virus Vaccines for Oral Immunisation of Wildlife

Several types of modified live-virus vaccines have been proposed for oral immunisation of animals in the past 20 years; however, only five have proved suitable for use in the field for vaccination of foxes (Canada and Europe) and raccoon dogs (Finland). All these vaccines are derivatives of the original SAD (Street Alabama Dufferin)-attenuated virus, which was isolated from a rabid dog in Alabama (USA) in 1935, then passaged in mouse brain cells (ERA strain) and adapted to BHK cells by various passages (SAD Berne) (Steck et al. 1982; WHO 2012; Cliquet 2012).

Four SAD-related vaccines (ERA, SAD-Bern, SAD-B19, and Vnukovo-32) are pathogenic for adult mice (by the intracerebral, intramuscular, and oral routes) and for many other rodent species. They do not appear to be pathogenic for North American and European carnivores and other large mammals when they are given by the oral route, except in the case of skunks (WHO 2012).

SAG vaccine is a deletion mutant of SAD developed using selected MAb. SAG vaccine is pathogenic neither for adult mice nor for any

Table 6.3 Some rabies veterinary vaccines available in India

Brand name, manufacturer, product detail	Use, dosage, site, route of administration, packing detail[a]
Raksharab (Indian Immunologicals Ltd.)	Use: for immunisation of dogs and other domestic animals against rabies, for prophylactic use, age 3 months and above
Inactivated rabies virus with a potency > 1.0 IU per dose. The virus is propagated in BHK-21 cell line, inactivated with an aziridine compound and concentrated. Aluminium hydroxide is added as an adjuvant	Dose and route: 1 ml, subcutaneous or intramuscular
	Primary vaccination: at age 3 months and above
	Revaccination: immunity is conferred for 36 months. However, annual vaccination is recommended in endemic areas
	Packing: single-dose vial (1 ml), multidose vial of five doses (5 ml), multidose vial of 10 doses (10 ml)
Defensor (Lincoln, Nebraska Estate, USA; marketed by Pfizer Ltd.)	Use: for vaccination of healthy dogs, cats, cattle, and sheep at 3 months of age or older as an aid in preventing rabies
Rabies vaccine, cell culture-grown, chemically inactivated virus, killed vaccine	Dose and route: 1 ml, intramuscular or subcutaneous
	Primary vaccination in healthy dogs and cats: a single dose at 3 months of age or older, a repeat dose 1 year later
	Revaccination: annual revaccination with a single dose
	Packing: single-dose vial (1 ml), multidose 10 ml vial
Nobivac Rabies (Intervet International by, Boxmeer, the Netherlands; marketed by Intervet India Pvt. Ltd.)	Use: for active immunisation of healthy dogs, cats, cattle, sheep, goats, ferrets, foxes, and horses and in principle all healthy mammals against rabies
Inactivated rabies vaccine, contains inactivated culture of Rabies virus, cloned out of strain Pasteur RIVM, virus is grown on BHK-21 clone CT cell line and inactivated with β-propiolactone, aqueous aluminium phosphate suspension	Dose and route: 1 ml, subcutaneous or intramuscular injection depending on species
	Vaccination scheme:
	Dogs and cats – primary vaccination at 3 months of age or above, revaccination every 3 years (annual revaccination recommended in endemic areas), intramuscular or subcutaneous route
	Cattle, horse, sheep, goat – primary vaccination at 6 months of age or above, revaccination every 2 years (annual revaccination recommended in endemic areas), intramuscular route
	Ferrets – primary vaccination at 3 months of age or above, revaccination every year, subcutaneous route
	Packing: single-dose vial (1 ml), multidose vial of 10 doses
Rabigen Mono (Virbac SA, France; marketed by Virbac Animal Health India Pvt. Ltd.)	Use: for active immunisation of dogs, cats, cattle, and horses and in principle all mammals against rabies
Inactivated (cell culture) antirabies vaccine, prepared from fixed Rabies vaccinal strain Pasteur VP12 grown on BHK cell line and inactivated with β-propiolactone, adjunction of AlOH as an adjuvant	Dose and route: 1 ml, in dogs and cats – subcutaneous or intramuscular route; in cattle and horses – intramuscular route
	Primary vaccination:
	Carnivores – a single injection from 3 months of age[b]
	Herbivores – single injection from 6 months of age[b]
	Revaccination: annual revaccination recommended
	Packing: single-dose vial (1 ml), multidose vial (10 ml)

[a]Based on the company's product information. Consult product literature, guidelines, and local regulations before use
[b]Primary vaccination can be administered at an earlier age, but then a repeat injection must be given at 3 or 6 months of age depending on species

wild rodents tested by the oral, intramuscular, or intracerebral routes; however, it is pathogenic for suckling mice when given by the intracerebral and oral routes (WHO 2012).

The SAG2 vaccine (Rabigen, Virbac Laboratories, France) is a modified live attenuated rabies virus vaccine registered in 27 countries of the EU (European Medicines Agency registration) for oral administration in baits to foxes and raccoon dogs (Anonymous 2008; Cliquet et al. 2012). The SAG2 virus strain was selected from SAD-Bern in a two-step process of amino acid mutation (Lafay et al. 1994; Cliquet et al. 2012). Tetracycline (150 mg per bait) was used as a biological marker to assess the bait consumption.

6.2.3 Recombinant Vaccines for Oral Immunisation of Wildlife

The development of recombinant DNA technology has initiated a new era in rabies control. Recombinant vaccines cannot exhibit residual pathogenicity caused by rabies because they contain only single non-virulent gene products. Newer vaccines include a vaccinia-rabies glycoprotein V-RG recombinant oral vaccine and a live adenovirus recombinant oral vaccine. These are available under the brand names Raboral V-RG® and ONRAB®), respectively. Raboral V-RG® (Merial) is licensed in the USA for ORV in coyotes (*Canis latrans*) and raccoons and is used under experimental licence in grey foxes (*Urocyon cinereoargenteus*). ONRAB® (Artemis Technologies Inc., Guelph, Ontario, Canada), consisting of a human adenovirus type 5 vector containing the ERA glycoprotein gene, is used under CFIA (Canadian Food Inspection Agency) experimental permit in Canada for control of rabies in skunks and raccoons. Studies have shown that ONRAB® may serve as an effective tool for raccoon rabies control (Rosatte 2011; Fehlner-Gardiner et al. 2012).

6.2.3.1 Potency Requirements

Minimum potency requirements for oral vaccines for immunisation of wild animals have not been generally established, although the median effective doses (ED_{50}) of various modified live-virus and recombinant vaccines are known. Testing of the efficacy of candidate vaccines for oral immunisation involves vaccinating sufficient numbers of target animals maintained under captive conditions and challenging these with the virus. Subsequently, the vaccine requires testing in field trials. Apart from estimating the ability of the vaccine to induce virus-neutralising antibodies in the target species, environmental stability tests are also necessary to demonstrate that vaccine potency is retained under field conditions (WHO 2012).

References

Anonymous (2008) Rabigen SAG2. European Medicines Agency. http://www.ema.europa.eu/ema/index.jsp?curl=pages/medicines/veterinary/medicines/000043/vet_med_000182.jsp&mid=WC0b01ac058008d7a8. Accessed 11 June 2012

Anonymous (2010) New treatment for rabies advances after successful phase 1 trial in India. Science Daily, 14 Sept 2010. http://www.sciencedaily.com/releases/2010/09/100914121501.htm. Accessed 5 July 2012

Anonymous (2012) Rabies antibody combination. Crucell. http://www.crucell.com/R_and_D-Clinical_Development-Rabies_Antibody_Product. Accessed 11 June 2012

APCRI (2009) Manual on rabies immunoglobulin (RIG) administration, 1st edn. Association for Prevention and Control of Rabies in India, Bangalore

Bonito RF, de Oliveira NM, Nishioka Sde A (2004) Adverse reactions associated with a Fuenzalida-Palacios rabies vaccine: a quasiexperimental study. Rev Soc Bras Med Trop 37:7–9

Cliquet F (2012) Oral vaccines used for rabies control programmes: types, storage, quality control and performance in different species. European Commission. http://ec.europa.eu/food/animal/diseases/eradication/rabies_pres_19.pdf. Accessed 18 June 2012

Cliquet F, Robardet E, Must K, Laine M, Peik K, Picard-Meyer E, Guiot AL, Niin E (2012) Eliminating rabies in Estonia. PLoS Negl Trop Dis 6(2):e1535. doi:10.1371/journal.pntd.0001535

Ertl HCJ (2009) Novel vaccines to human rabies. PLoS Negl Trop Dis 3(9):e515. doi:10.1371/journal.pntd.0000515

Fehlner-Gardiner C, Rudd R, Donovan D, Slate D, Kempf L, Badcock J (2012) Comparing ONRAB® and RABORAL V-RG® oral rabies vaccine field performance in raccoons and striped skunks, New Brunswick, Canada, and Maine, USA. J Wildl Dis 48(1):157–167

Fernandes A, Kaundinya JO, Daftary G, Saxena L, Banerjee S, Pattnaik P (2008) Chromatographic purification of equine immunoglobulin G F(ab)2 from plasma. J Chromatogr B 876:109–115

Fox JP, Koprowski H, Conwell DP, Black J, Gelfand HM (1957) Study of antirabies immunization of man. Observations with HEP Flury and other vaccines, with and without hyperimmune serum, in primary and recall immunizations. Bull WHO 17:869–904

Fuenzalida E, Palacios R, Borgono JM (1964) Antirabies antibody responses in man to vaccine made from infected suckling-mouse brains. Bull WHO 30:431–436

Hicks DJ, Fooks AR, Johnson N (2012) Developments in rabies vaccines. Clin Exp Immunol. doi:10.1111/j.1365-2249.2012.04592.x

Kittipongwarakarn S, Hawe A, Tantipolphan R, Limsuwun K, Khomvilai S, Puttipipatkhachorn S, Jiskoot W (2011) New method to produce equine antirabies immunoglobulin F(ab')2 fragments from crude plasma in high quality and yield. Eur J Pharm Biopharm 78:189–195

Koprowski L, Cox HR (1948) Studies on chick embryo adapted rabies virus: I Culture characteristics and pathogenicity. J Immunol 60:533–554

Lafay F, Benejean J, Tuffereau C, Flamand A, Coulon P (1994) Vaccination against rabies: construction and characterization of SAG2, a double avirulent derivative of SADBern. Vaccine 12:317–320

Leach CN, Johnson HN (1940) Human rabies, with special reference to virus distribution and titer. Am J Trop Med Hyg 20:335–340

Mahendra BJ, Madhusudana SN, Sampath G, Datta SS, Ashwathnarayana DH, Venkatesh GM, Sudarshan MK, Bilugumba G, Shamanna M (2010) Immunogenicity, safety and tolerance of a purified duck embryo vaccine (PDEV, VAXIRAB) for rabies post-exposure prophylaxis – results of a multicentric study in India. Hum Vaccine 6(9):721–724

McGettigan JP (2010) Experimental rabies vaccines for humans. Expert Rev Vaccines 9:1177–1186. doi:10.1586/erv.10.105

Müller T, Dietzschold B, Ertl H, Fooks AR, Freuling C, Fehlner-Gardiner C, Kliemt J, Meslin FX, Rupprecht CE, Tordo N, Wanderler AI, Kieny MP (2009) Development of a mouse monoclonal antibody cocktail for post-exposure rabies prophylaxis in humans. PLoS Negl Trop Dis 3(11):e542. doi:10.1371/journal.pntd.0000542

Nandi S, Kumar M (2010) Development in immunoprophylaxis against rabies for animals and humans. Avicenna J Med Biotechnol 2(1):3–21

Peck FB, Powell HM, Culbertson CG (1955) A new antirabies vaccine for human use. Appl Microbiol 45:679–683

Ramya R, Mohana Subramanian B, Sivakumar V, Senthilkumar RL, Sambasiva Rao KRS, Srinivasan VA (2011) Expression and solubilization of insect cell-based rabies virus glycoprotein and assessment of its immunogenicity and protective efficacy in mice. Clin Vaccine Immunol 18:1673–1679. doi:10.1128/CVI.05258-11

Rosatte R (2011) Evolution of wildlife rabies control tactics. Adv Virus Res 79:397–419

Semple D (1911) The preparation of a safe and efficient antirabic vaccine. Sci Mem Med Sanit Dept India 44:1–31

Steck F, Wandeler A, Bischel P, Hafliger U, Schneider L (1982) Oral immunisation of foxes against rabies. Laboratory and field studies. Comp Immunol Microbiol Infect Dis 5:165–171

Sveshnikov PG, Yagudin TA, Morozkina EV, Klyachko EV, Zatsepin SS, Benevolensky SV, Shemchukova OB, Pozdnyakova LP, Solopova ON (2010) Production of a humanized Fab fragment of a neutralizing antibody against rabies virus. Moscow Univ Chem Bull 65:154–158. doi:10.3103/S0027131410030090

Ullas PT, Desai A, Madhusudana SN (2012) Rabies DNA vaccines: current status and future. World J Vaccines 2:36–45. doi:10.4236/wjv.2012.21005

Vodopija I, Clarke HF (1991) Human vaccination against rabies. In: Baer GM (ed) The natural history of rabies, 2nd edn. CRC Press, Boca Raton, pp 571–595

WHO (1981) Requirements for rabies vaccine for human use. WHO Expert Committee on Biological Standardization. Thirty-first report. WHO technical report series, no. 658, Annex 2. World Health Organization, Geneva

WHO (1987) Requirements for rabies vaccine (inactivated) for human use produced in continuous cell lines. WHO Expert Committee on Biological Standardization. Thirty-seventh report. WHO technical report series, no. 760. World Health Organization, Geneva

WHO (1994a) Requirements for rabies vaccine for human use. WHO Expert Committee on Biological Standardization. Forty-third report. WHO technical report series, no. 840, Annex 4. World Health Organization, Geneva

WHO (1994b) Requirements for rabies vaccine (inactivated) for human use produced in continuous cell lines. WHO Expert Committee on Biological Standardization. Forty-third report. WHO technical report series, no. 840, Annex 5. World Health Organization, Geneva

WHO (2007) Recommendations for inactivated rabies vaccine for human use produced in cell substrates and embryonated eggs. WHO Expert Committee on Biological Standardization. Fifty-sixth report. WHO technical report series, no. 941, Annex 2. World Health Organization, Geneva

WHO (2010) Rabies vaccines: WHO position paper. Wkly Epidemiol Rec No 32 85:309–320

WHO (2012) Rabies. World Health Organization. www.who.int. Accessed 10 Mar 2012

WHO SEARO (2012) Rabies: Country profile: India. World Health Organization, Regional Office for South-East Asia, New Delhi. http://www.searo.who.int/LinkFiles/Zoonoses_IND-rabies-cp.pdf. Accessed 15 Aug 2012

Wu X, Franka R, Henderson H, Rupprecht CE (2011a) Live attenuated rabies virus co-infected with street rabies virus protects animals against rabies. Vaccine 29:4195–4201

Wu X, Smith TG, Rupprecht CE (2011b) From brain passage to cell adaptation: the road of human rabies vaccine development. Expert Rev Vaccines 10:1597–1608

Rabies Prevention and Control

7

Abstract

Despite its severity and high incidence, rabies continues to be largely neglected in the developing world. Multiplex strategies are required for rabies control in animals and humans. Effective national plans need to be evolved by the rabies-affected countries taking cue from the countries which have been able to successfully control or even eliminate the disease. Since the best way of prevention of rabies is to avoid rabies exposure, reduction of stray dog population and elimination of rabies in dogs constitute the mainstay of any rabies control programme. Mass educational campaigns and legislative measures are important in seeking public support. The Animal Welfare Board of India is promoting the implementation of Animal Birth Control (ABC) and Anti-Rabies (AR) programme in the country. The countries facing the problem of sylvatic rabies need to control the disease in wildlife reservoirs. Provision of prompt medical care and postexposure prophylactic immunisation is essential to protect the persons exposed to infection. A number of factors and constraints that may obstruct the action plans have been elaborated in this chapter.

7.1 Prevention and Control Strategies

Despite its severity and high incidence in developing countries, rabies continues to be largely a neglected disease. Though a variety of animal reservoirs are known to transmit rabies to human beings, dogs constitute by far the most common cause of human rabies infections in the world. It is quite evident that the rabies transmission cycle can be broken only through prevention and control of rabies in animal source. As dog is the principal reservoir of rabies, particularly in the developing countries, eliminating rabies in dogs is the most important approach for rabies prevention and control. Multiplex strategies are required for successful and sustainable rabies control in animals and humans. These have been elaborated by Garg (2012) and briefly outlined below.

7.1.1 Evolving a Comprehensive Rabies Control Programme

Rabies prevention and control programmes have led to successful control or even elimination

S.R. Garg, *Rabies in Man and Animals*, DOI 10.1007/978-81-322-1605-6_7,

of rabies in several countries or regions including the developing nations. Taking cue from their operational strategies and experiences, appropriate national plans for rabies control should be evolved by the rabies-affected countries. An Interregional Consultation organised by the World Health Organization in Geneva in 2001 has recommended inclusion of the following components in the national plans (WHO 2001):

- Access to modern human vaccines and application of new economical postexposure prophylaxis (PEP)
- Rabies surveillance and collection and processing of data at the national, regional, and global levels
- Intersectoral collaborative efforts for controlling rabies in dogs at national and regional levels
- Plan to increase the awareness concerning rabies control and prevention among the public and healthcare workers
- A detailed budget covering a 3- to 5-year period
- A time frame and targets for each year

It has been recommended that political commitment and leadership for the national plan should be through the Ministry of Health, with additional partnerships that are appropriate to implement the programme within each country. While the health department is mainly responsible for prevention of rabies in human beings, veterinary services are responsible for regulation of rabies control programmes in dogs and other animals. The support of many other relevant national departments and agencies is also inevitable. These include departments of finance, education, internal home affairs, law and justice, municipalities, village *panchayats*, municipal councils, district councils, and academic and research institutions (e.g. faculties of Veterinary Sciences and Human Medicine). It is also essential to rope in the non-governmental organisations (NGOs), private sector, and media in the programme for its success. International agencies such as the WHO, OIE, FAO, PAHO, and worldwide veterinary associations provide guidelines and support for the provision and supply of appropriate biologicals for national and regional planning of rabies control programmes (Partners for Rabies Prevention 2010).

A rabies elimination programme funded by the Gates Foundation and coordinated by the WHO was launched in the Richards Bay/Uthungulu area of KwaZulu-Natal province in South Africa in April 2011. Two similar programmes funded by Gates Foundation are running in Tanzania and the Philippines.

India, despite carrying the maximum burden of rabies, does not have a comprehensive National Rabies Control Programme. However, a pilot project on prevention and control of human rabies was initiated in January 2008 in five cities, viz., Ahmedabad, Bangalore, Pune, Delhi, and Madurai. The project focused on the training of health professionals in animal bite management, wider coverage of PEP, availability of adequate and cost-effective vaccines and rabies immunoglobulin (RIG), implementation of intradermal route for vaccination, enhancing awareness about timely and adequate postexposure treatment in the community, sensitisation of veterinarians, and strengthening of diagnostic capabilities and surveillance (Mittal 2009; WHO SEARO 2012).

India has vast medical, paramedical, and veterinary professional human resource. The country also has the capability to produce enough modern antirabies vaccines and RIG. A large number of dedicated scientific societies and NGOs are already working for rabies control, and the Animal Welfare Board of India (AWBI) has been providing support for the Animal Birth Control and Anti-Rabies (ABC-AR) programme in many parts of the country. However, it is desirable to bring all the stakeholders to a common platform, build consensus, establish intersectoral coordination, and evolve a comprehensive programme for the country. The Association for Prevention and Control of Rabies in India (APCRI) recommended launching of such programme long back using the approaches given in Box 7.1 (APCRI 2006). The Government of India is in the active process of launching a nationwide rabies control programme.

Box 7.1 Approaches for Rabies Control (APCRI 2006)

- Human rabies prevention
  - Postexposure prophylaxis (PEP)
  - Pre-exposure prophylaxis
  - Advancement of diagnostics
- Maintaining rabies-free areas
  - Maintaining rabies-free status of the rabies-free areas
  - Monitoring and surveillance
- Animal reservoir control
  - Control of community dog population
  - Compulsory vaccination and licensing of pet dogs
  - Mass parenteral annual vaccination of community dogs

7.1.2 Prompt Management of Animal Bite Wounds

The best way of prevention of possible exposures to rabies virus is to avoid animal bites (mainly dogs, monkeys, bats, cats, and wild animals). Licks from animals to fresh wounds or mucous membranes should also be avoided to ward off the possibility of exposure. However, accidental exposures are not uncommon. In India alone, the annual animal bite incidence has been estimated at 17.4 million cases in a year (APCRI 2004). Bite wound care can substantially reduce the risk of infection. Animal bite or scratch should receive prompt care and management because immediate and adequate medical care is critical to preventing rabies.

7.1.3 Improving Access to Modern Cell Culture Vaccines

Prompt PEP significantly reduces the number of human rabies cases. It is estimated that about 327,000 persons would die from rabies in Africa and Asia each year in the absence of PEP (Knobel et al. 2005). Modern purified cell culture and embryonated egg-based rabies vaccines are safe and effective in pre-exposure prophylaxis as well as PEP against rabies (WHO 2010). Modern vaccines are much better than the nerve tissue vaccines which are less immunogenic and bear the risk of inducing adverse reactions.

India has stopped producing and using nerve tissue vaccine (Semple vaccine produced in sheep) since 2005 and has replaced it with modern vaccines. However, cell culture vaccines are much expensive in comparison to the nerve tissue vaccines, limiting their access and use particularly in less-developed countries. Probably due to this reason, many countries, mainly in Asia and Latin America, still depend on rabies vaccines derived from animal nerve tissues for PEP (WHO 2010). In India too, Semple vaccine was earlier freely available in government hospitals, but the availability of cell culture vaccines is not as good due to budgetary constraints. The cost of one dose of cell culture rabies vaccine is about Rs. 350, making the full course of five doses by intramuscular route quite expensive for the animal bite victims who are generally poor. Moreover, the modern vaccines may not be easily available in rural and remote areas leading to delay in initiating the PEP immunisation. Easy access to modern vaccines is very crucial in protecting the patients from the grave risk of contracting rabies.

7.1.4 Promoting Timely and Adequate Immunisation

Postexposure treatment should start immediately wherever recommended according to the prescribed guidelines. Factors that should be taken into consideration when deciding whether to initiate PEP include the epidemiological likelihood of the implicated animal being rabid, the category of exposure, and the clinical features of the animal as well as its availability for observation and laboratory testing. Many times the information about the PEP vaccination status of the implicated animal may not be reliable; hence it may not be advisable to withhold PEP even if the animal is vaccinated (WHO 2010).

PEP involves administration of antirabies vaccine and depending upon the exposure category, application of RIG. Strict adherence to the complete vaccination regimen and administration of vaccine by the prescribed route and at recommended site are important for the success of the immunisation process. Where administration of RIG is also required along with vaccination, vaccination alone may not be sufficient for protection. Skipping of RIG administration in such cases may lead to prophylaxis failure.

7.1.5 Promoting Cost-Effective Intradermal Vaccination

Full course of PEP vaccination by the intramuscular route is quite expensive, which generally limits its use, particularly in the developing countries where canine rabies is widespread. Intradermal administration of cell culture vaccines offers an equally safe and immunogenic alternative that requires less amount of vaccine, resulting in considerably reduced cost of a full course of vaccination. However in certain settings where sufficient number of patients is not available for vaccination, the reconstituted leftover vaccine is expected to be wasted. The provision of specially pre-packaged vaccine vials for intradermal use may help in preventing wastage and cost-effectiveness of the expensive biological.

7.1.6 Evolving More Efficient Cost-Effective Biologicals

Rabies deaths can be substantially reduced by increasing the availability and accessibility of antirabies vaccines and RIG. While it is important to make provision for adequate availability of rabies biologicals, avoiding their wastage and unnecessary use is also equally important in view of the high costs and the limited supply. Development of new cost-effective rabies biologicals and antiviral drugs is critical in continuing to prevent and reduce the disease. Current rabies vaccines are highly effective but alternative approaches for improved vaccines, including novel avirulent rabies virus vectors, should be pursued (Smith et al. 2011). Development of rabies vaccine that is fully protective without the need for RIG can substantially bring down the cost and complexity of PEP. Virus-specific monoclonal antibody (MAb) should be evolved for providing passive immunity, replacing the currently available expensive and generally unaffordable RIG.

7.1.7 Vaccination of Dogs

Vaccination of dogs and elimination of rabies in dogs constitute the mainstay of any rabies control programme. It provides a more cost-effective and efficient tool with long-term benefits than the post-bite treatment of individual cases. The cost of a post-bite treatment in humans is about 20–100 times more than the vaccination of a dog (OIE 2009). Thus, veterinary services would be able to eradicate rabies in animals and consequently stop almost all human cases with only 10 % of the financial resources used worldwide to treat people after a dog bite.

Many industrialised countries either have eliminated or are close to elimination of human rabies through vaccination of domestic dogs and implementation of other control measures. The developing countries should also develop on high priority the strategies for canine vaccination. They should organise mass dog vaccination programmes in a planned manner (Figs. 7.1 and 7.2).

7.1.8 Evolving Oral Rabies Vaccination

Administration of vaccination by the parenteral route to stray dogs is a tedious process requiring huge manpower and financial resources. It makes the task of covering sufficient numbers of dogs in an area speedily very difficult creating problem in attaining the desirable level of vaccinated dog population in an area at a time. This is particularly so in the countries with large population of stray or unsupervised dogs. Development of safe and effective oral vaccines may help in mass vaccination of animals in a wide area.

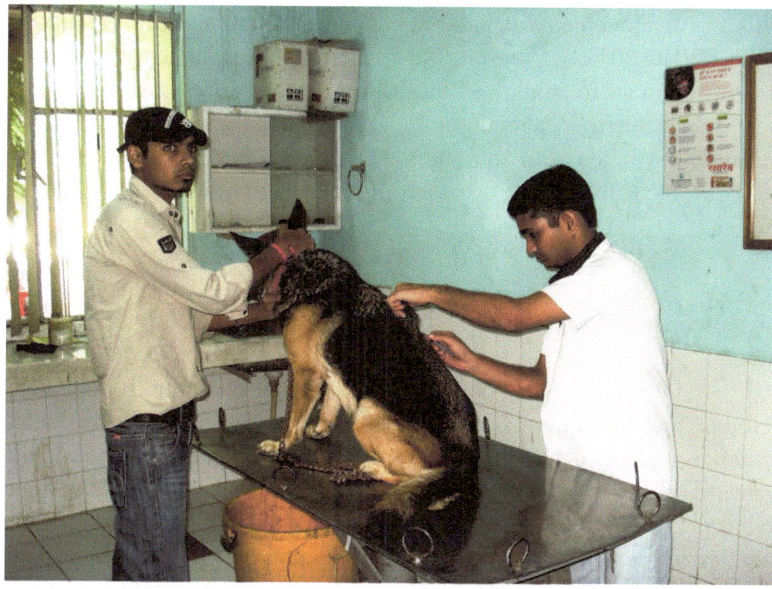

Fig. 7.1 Antirabies vaccination in a pet dog

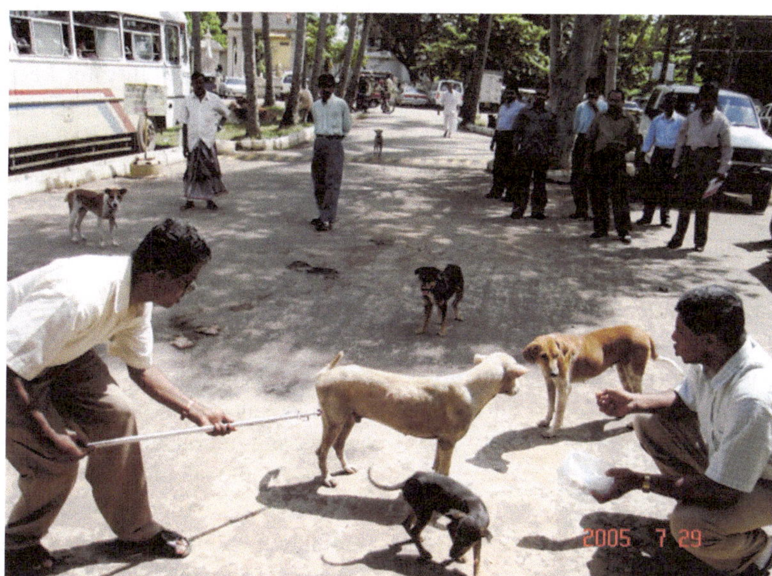

Fig. 7.2 Stray dog vaccination in Sri Lanka (Photo Credit: Dr. P. A. L. Harischandra)

7.1.9 Managing Dog Population

Apart from mass vaccination of dogs, reduction of unsupervised stray dog population is also important in the countries where dog rabies is prevalent. It has been observed that indiscriminate mass culling and destruction of dogs may not bring the desired results in rabies control. There is no evidence that removal of dogs alone has ever had a significant impact on dog population densities or the spread of rabies but targeted and humane removal of unvaccinated, ownerless dogs may be effective when used as a supplementary measure to mass vaccination (WHO 2012a). Dog removal and destruction being contrary to animal welfare may however be unacceptable to local communities. Mass sterilisation combined with antirabies vaccination is thus a practicable result-oriented approach.

7.1.10 Strengthening of Laboratory Facilities

Laboratory facilities are important for rapid diagnosis of the disease, quality assurance of biologicals, and evaluation of the immunity development. These facilities help in timely initiation and success of the rabies prophylaxis. Laboratory facilities also help in evaluation of duration of immunity of the vaccination, thus facilitating optimal application and utilisation of rabies biologicals.

7.1.11 Strengthening of Rabies Surveillance System

Epidemiological surveillance involves estimation of incidence and prevalence of disease in a geographical region. Strengthening of rabies surveillance and data collection systems is essential to determine the most affected areas and other epidemiological features of the disease. The information provides the foundation for planning rabies control measures and also to demonstrate the effectiveness of such programmes.

7.1.12 Mass Education

Lack of awareness among the people about rabies, the risks associated with the disease, and the action to be taken in the event of an exposure is a major reason for the occurrence of the disease in man and animals. In a multi-country survey conducted by the Asian Rabies Expert Bureau (AREB) in Bangladesh, China, India, Indonesia, Pakistan, the Philippines, Sri Lanka, and Thailand, it has been observed that in the instances of rabies exposure, people's awareness of the necessity to apply appropriate wound care and to consult the nearest rabies prevention centre as soon as possible can make a big difference in the rabies situation in the world (Dodet et al. 2008). Mass educational campaigns are important. These assume the greatest importance in the developing countries like India, where sizeable population is illiterate, semiliterate, and less informed (Figs. 7.3 and 7.4). People need to be educated about the wound care practices and importance of seeking medical help immediately instead of wasting time in home remedies after an animal bite. They need to be emphatically told that the delays in starting or failure to complete correct prophylaxis may result in death, particularly after being bitten in highly innervated regions, such as head, neck, or hands, or when there are multiple wounds (Wilde 2007).

People's participation is paramount for the success of a rabies prevention and control programme. Mass education programmes should promote responsible dog ownership at the community level. Pet owners should be educated about their responsibility for keeping the movements of their pets restricted and supervised. They should also be instructed to follow the rules of pet animal registration and vaccination guidelines. Dog owners should be guided to restrict the movement of their pets. They should be educated to prevent the risk caused by their pets to the people, other pets, livestock, and wildlife. They should be made responsible for the hazards caused by their pets. Legal mechanisms are necessary to deal with irresponsible owners and imposition of penalties.

The people should be pursued to provide full cooperation to the agencies involved in dog population management and rabies control by desisting from feeding stray animals, avoiding garbage disposal in open, and participating in the vaccination campaigns.

7.1.13 Enforcing Legislative Measures

Legislative measures such as tie-up orders, individual animal identification, and pet animal registration are necessary to enforce responsible

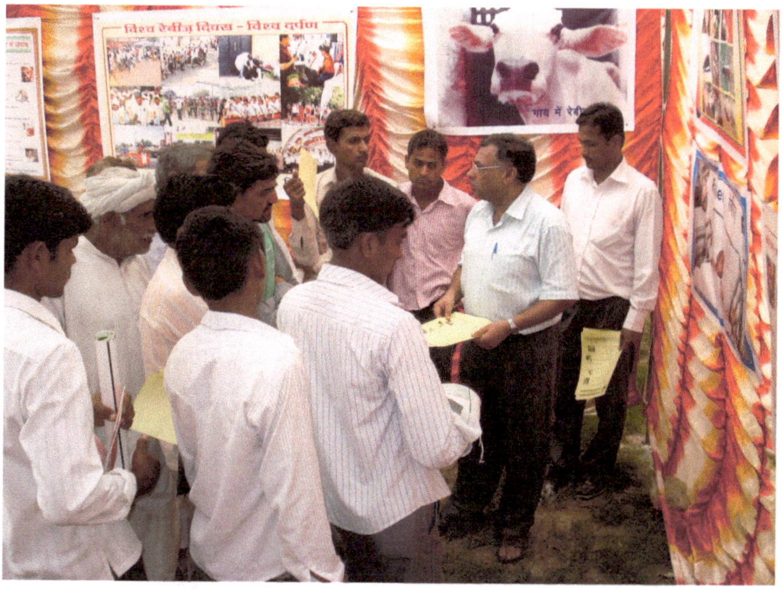

Fig. 7.3 The author interacting with people in a mass rabies awareness campaign

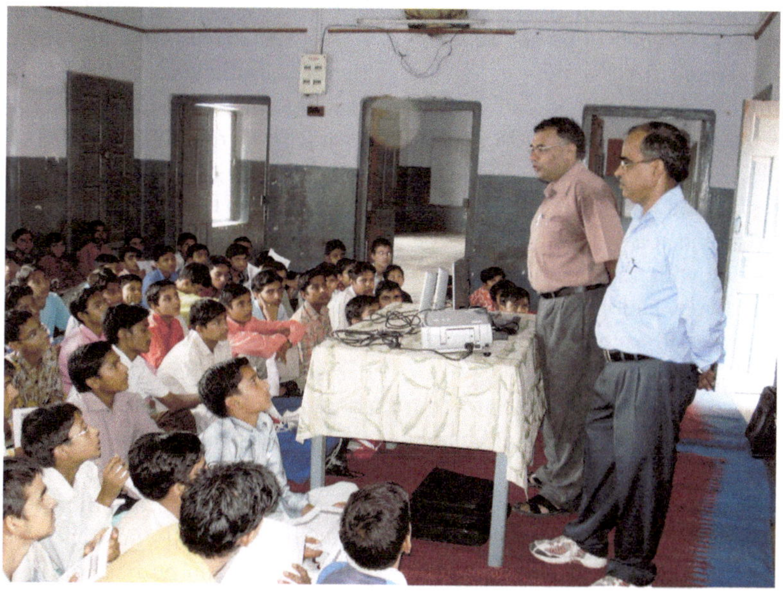

Fig. 7.4 The author interacting with schoolchildren regarding rabies prevention

pet ownership. Border checks, control of pet animal trade, restriction on animal movements, and other measures should be implemented to prevent the introduction of rabies into rabies-free areas (Partners for Rabies Prevention 2010). There should be strict laws and regulations concerning companion animal travel, animal importation, and animal trade to avoid spread and reintroduction of the disease, particularly in those countries which are rabies-free. During transborder movement, animals should have proper identification, complete documentation, and valid rabies vaccination certificate. In addition, a laboratory report of rabies antibody titre in the blood may also be obtained.

Making it mandatory to notify the cases of rabies and animal bites is also important. It can facilitate surveillance, estimation of disease burden, and evolving rational and result-oriented disease control strategies.

7.2 Stray Dog Population Control

Stray and feral dogs pose serious human health, animal health, and animal welfare problems and have a socio-economic, environmental, political, and religious impact in many countries (OIE 2011). Dog population management is an integral part of rabies control programmes.

7.2.1 Types of Dogs

A dog for which a person claims responsibility may be treated as an owned dog, but any dog not under direct control of a person or not prevented from roaming is considered a stray dog. A stray dog may belong to any of the following categories:

- Free-roaming owned dog not under direct control or restriction at a particular time
- Free-roaming dog with no owner
- Feral dog, i.e. domestic dog that has reverted to the wild state and is no longer directly dependent upon humans

In India, dogs can be distributed into four categories based on their dependence on humans and their movements:

1. Restricted or supervised owned pet dogs – These are wholly dependent on owners and the movements of these dogs are restricted by the pet owners.
2. Family dogs – These are wholly dependent on humans, but their movements are only partially restricted by the owners.
3. Neighbourhood or community dogs – These are partially dependent on humans (community), but their movements are wholly unrestricted.
4. Feral dogs – These are independent or depend on human waste/garbage alone. Their movements are completely unrestricted.

A vast majority of dogs belong to the last three categories in India. The unrestricted movements of dogs not only make them vulnerable to infection but also increase the transmission of rabies to humans.

7.2.2 Dog Population Control Programme

Dog population control programme means a programme with the aim of reducing a stray dog population to a particular level and/or maintaining it at that level and/or managing it in order to meet a predetermined objective. According to the OIE Terrestrial Animal Health Code (OIE 2011), such a programme may include the following objectives:

1. Reduction in the numbers of stray dogs to an acceptable level
2. Improvement in health and welfare of owned and stray dog population
3. Promotion of responsible ownership
4. Assistance in creating and maintaining a rabies immune or rabies-free dog population
5. Reduction of the risk of zoonotic diseases other than rabies
6. Prevention of health risks to other animals
7. Prevention of environmental degradation
8. Prevention of illegal trade and trafficking of animals

OIE (2011) recommends that while developing a dog population control programme, the authorities should establish an advisory group, which should include veterinarians; experts in dog ecology, dog behaviour, and zoonotic diseases; and representatives of the local authorities, human health services/authorities, environmental control services/authorities, NGOs, and the public. The main purpose of this advisory group would be to analyse and quantify the problem, identify the causes, obtain public opinion on dogs, and propose the most effective approaches to use in the short and long term.

7.2.3 Methods of Stray Dog Control

OIE has laid down recommendations to deal with stray dog population control (OIE 2011).

The guiding principles for these recommendations include:

- Dog population control should be done without causing unnecessary animal suffering.
- Promoting responsible dog ownership can significantly reduce the numbers of stray dogs and the incidence of zoonotic diseases.
- Along with dog population control, changes in human behaviour are also required because dog ecology is linked with human activities.

A number of stray dog control strategies described by the OIE (2011) are briefly summarised below. These can be implemented according to the national context and local circumstances and may be used in combination. Euthanasia of dogs, used alone, is not an effective control measure. If used, it should be done humanely and in combination with other measures to achieve effective long-term control (OIE 2011). Attempts to control dog populations through culling, without alteration of habitat and resource availability, have generally been unsuccessful.

7.2.3.1 Education and Legislation for Responsible Ownership

The promotion of responsible dog ownership through education and legislation is a necessary part of a dog population control programme. They should also be educated about proper selection and care of a dog, proper socialisation and training of the dog, registration and identification of dogs, and disease prevention through regular vaccination in rabies-endemic areas. Mandatory registration and identification of owned dogs is important to ensure responsible pet ownership, effective animal health programmes, rabies vaccination, and traceability. Pet owners should also be told to control reproduction of pets according to their carrying capacity based on availability of resources (food, water, shelter) and human acceptance for the welfare of their pets, their own families, as well as the community.

7.2.3.2 Reproductive Control

Controlling reproduction in dogs prevents disproportionate growth of dog population. Sterilisation of dogs requires involvement of veterinary services, in both the public and private sectors. Funding from the government or other organisations is essential for the reproductive control programmes.

7.2.3.3 Capture and Removal of Stray Dogs

It involves capturing and removal of stray dogs from an area. The staff should be adequately trained to carry out the job of dog capture, transport, handling, and holding in a humane manner. Appropriate legislation and availability of proper equipment are also important for humane handling of the animals.

7.2.3.4 Capture and Return, Rehoming, or Release

In this approach, dogs that are removed from a community may be reunited with the owners or offered to new owners for rehoming. However, the scope of rehoming is very limited due to poor acceptance of such abandoned or stray dogs and also due to their large numbers. The dogs after sterilisation and rabies vaccination can be released back to the place or a nearby place from where these were captured if it is permissible by law and acceptable to the local community. In other instances, it is required to make provision of adequate shelter, food, water, healthcare services, etc. for holding and maintaining such dogs. If euthanasia of these unwanted animals is the only option, the procedure should be carried out humanely and in accordance with the regulations.

7.2.3.5 Habitat Control

Dog population can be controlled by preventing their access to the sources of food and garbage. It can be achieved by holding the waste in animal-proof enclosures or containers. Protection of slaughterhouse waste is particularly important.

7.2.3.6 Control of Transborder and Inland Dog Movement

Transborder movement, export, and import of dogs should be guided by the legislative provisions. Similarly, movement of dogs within a country or an area can be controlled by local laws putting restrictions on unsupervised unleashed movement of dogs.

7.2.3.7 Regulation of Commercial Dog Dealers

A regulatory mechanism should be evolved for dog breeders and dealers so that they observe good practices for raising healthy animals in proper conditions and under veterinary supervision. They should be asked to raise and sell physically and psychologically healthy dogs and provide guidance to the new pet owners about proper care of their pets, as unhealthy dogs may be more likely to be abandoned to become part of the stray population.

7.2.3.8 Euthanasia

When euthanasia is practised, approved humane methods should be used to minimise distress, anxiety, and pain to the animals according to the general principles in the Terrestrial Code and local legislations. The operators should be properly trained and their safety should be ensured. In India, the Animal Birth Control (Dogs) Rules, 2001, have a provision of humanely euthanising dogs under certain circumstances (GOI 2001). Incurably sick, mortally wounded or rabid dogs may be euthanised as per these rules. The dogs found to be extremely aggressive and bad tempered, prone to biting people, and with a history of having bitten people may also be included in this category (AWBI 2009).

The method of euthanasia should be painless. It should achieve rapid unconsciousness followed by death with minimal animal fear and distress. The method should be reliable and irreversible. According to the AWBI guidelines, in India, euthanasia should be carried out using intravenous injection of 20 % solution of thiopentone sodium (90 mg/kg bodyweight) after sedation with xylazine. Alternatively 10 % potassium chloride can be used as a euthanising agent after xylazine sedation (AWBI 2009). Confirmation of death after the procedure is essential and all operators should be able to identify when death has occurred.

7.2.4 Methods of Reproduction Control

Dog reproduction control involves catching, neutering, and releasing the dogs in their original habitats by the civic bodies. The rationale of reproduction control is to reduce the dog population turnover as well as the number of dogs susceptible to rabies and influence the male dog behaviour such as dispersal and fighting, which otherwise facilitate the spread of rabies (WHO 2005).

The control of unwanted reproduction of dogs can be achieved by surgical sterilisation, chemical sterilisation, or chemical contraception. Separation of female dogs during oestrus from unsterilised males also helps (OIE 2011). Surgical sterilisation should be carried out by a veterinarian and includes appropriate anaesthesia and pain management. Any chemicals or drugs used in controlling reproduction should be shown to have appropriate safety, quality, and efficacy for the function required, and these should be used according to the manufacturer's instructions and the competent authority's regulations. In case of chemical sterilants and contraceptives, research and field trials may need to be completed before use.

7.2.5 Animal Birth Control Rules in India

Animal birth control programmes coupled with rabies vaccination have been advocated as a method to control dog populations and ultimately human rabies in Asia since the 1960s (WHO 2005). The Government of India notified the Animal Birth Control (Dogs) Rules, 2001 (ABC Rules), in the year 2001 under the Prevention of Cruelty to Animals Act, 1960. The principal rules were published in the Gazette of India on December 24, 2001 (GOI 2001). Later, some amendments were made through Animal Birth Control (Dogs) Amendment Rules, 2010, that were notified on February 8, 2011, by the Ministry of Environment and Forests, Government of India (GOI 2011). The scope and main features of the ABC Rules are briefly summarised below.

7.2.5.1 Classification of Dogs and Their Sterilisation

1. According to the ABC Rules, all dogs shall be classified in one of the following two categories: (i) pet dogs and (ii) street dogs.

2. The owner of pet dogs shall be responsible for the controlled breeding, immunisation, sterilisation, and licensing in accordance with the ABC Rules and the law for the time being in force within a specified local area.
3. The street dogs shall be sterilised and immunised by participation of animal welfare organisations, private individuals, and the local authority.

7.2.5.2 Formation of Committee

A monitoring committee consisting of the following persons shall be constituted by the local authority, for a period of 3 years, namely, Commissioner/Chief of the local authority, who shall be the ex officio Chairman of the committee, a representative of the Public Health Department of the local authority, representative of the Animal Welfare Department if any of the local authority, a veterinary doctor, a representative of the District Society for Prevention of Cruelty to Animals (SPCA), at least two representatives from the Animal Welfare Organizations operating within the said local authority, and a representative of the people who is a humanitarian or a well-known individual who has experience in animal welfare in the locality.

7.2.5.3 Functions of the Committee

The committee constituted as above shall be responsible for planning and management of dog control programme in accordance with the ABC Rules. The committee may:

a. Issue instructions for catching, transportation, sheltering, sterilisation, vaccination, treatment, and release of sterilised vaccinated or treated dogs.
b. Authorise the veterinary doctor to decide on case-to-case basis the need to put to sleep critically ill or fatally injured or rabid dogs in a painless manner by using sodium pentothal. Any other method is strictly prohibited.
c. Create public awareness and solicit cooperation and funding.
d. Provide guidelines to pet dog owners and commercial breeders from time to time.
e. Get a survey done of the number of street dogs by an independent agency.
f. Take such steps for monitoring the dog bite cases to ascertain the reasons of dog bite, the area where it took place, and whether it was from a stray or a pet dog.
g. Keep a watch on the national and international development in the field of research pertaining to street dogs control and management, development of vaccines, and cost-effective methods of sterilisation, vaccination, etc.

The ABC Rules require that the activities of the committee shall be brought to the public notice by announcements and advertisements.

7.2.5.4 Obligations of the Local Authority

The obligations of the local authority envisaged in the ABC Rules are summarised below.

1. The local authority shall provide for:
   (a) Establishment of a sufficient number of dog pounds including animal kennels/shelters which may be managed by animal welfare organisations
   (b) Requisite number of dog vans with ramps for the capture and transportation of street dogs
   (c) One driver and two trained dog catchers for each dog van
   (d) An ambulance cum clinical van as mobile centre for sterilisation and immunisation
   (e) Incinerators for disposal of carcasses
   (f) Periodic repair of shelter or pound
2. If the Municipal Corporation or the local authority thinks it expedient to control street dog population, it shall be incumbent upon them to sterilise and immunise street dogs with the participation of animal welfare organisations, private individuals, and the local authority.
3. The animal welfare organisations shall be reimbursed the expenses of sterilisation/immunisation at a rate to be fixed by the committee on fortnightly basis based on the number of sterilisation/immunisation done.
4. The monitoring committee of the said locality shall meet at least once in every month to assess the progress made in regard to implementation of the ABC Programme.

7.2.5.5 Capturing/Sterilisation/ Immunisation/Release

The ABC Rules provide as below:

1. Capturing of dogs shall be based on:
   (a) Specific complaints (for which the local authority in consultation with the monitoring committee shall set up a dog control cell to receive complaints about dog nuisance, dog bites, and information about rabid dogs)
   (b) General
      (i) On receipt of specific complaint about nuisance or dog bite, the same shall be attended on priority basis, irrespective of the area from which the complaint comes. On receipt of such complaint, the details such as name of the complainant, his complete address, date and time of complaint, and nature of complaint shall be recorded in a register to be maintained for permanent record.
      (ii) Capturing for general purpose will be on such dates and time to be specified by the committee.
2. The dog-capturing squad shall consist of driver of the dog van, two or more trained employees of the local authority who are trained in capturing of dogs, and one representative of any of the animal welfare organisation.

   Each member of the dog squad shall carry a valid identity card issued by the local authority. The dog-capturing squad will be accompanied by a representative of an animal welfare organisation nominated for the purpose.
3. On receipt of specific complaint or for capturing dogs in normal course, the dog squad will visit the concerned area and capture the dogs identified by the complaint in case of complaint-oriented capturing and other dogs in case of general capturing. All the dogs caught will be tagged for identification purposes and to ensure that the dogs are released in the same area after sterilisation and vaccination. Only stipulated number of dogs, according to the ABC Programme target, shall be caught by the van. A record of dogs captured shall be maintained in a register, mentioning therein the name of the area/locality, date and time of capture, names of persons in the dog squad on that particular day, and details about dogs captured such as number of male dogs, number of female dogs, and number of puppies.
4. The dogs shall be captured by using humane methods such as lassoing or soft-loop animal catchers such as those prescribed under the provisions of Prevention of Cruelty (Capture of Animals) Rules, 1979.
5. While dogs are being captured in any locality, the representative of the local authority or of the animal welfare organisation accompanying the dog squad will make announcements on a public address system that dogs are being captured from the area for the purpose of sterilisation and immunisation and will be released in the same area after sterilisation and immunisation. The announcement may also briefly educate the residents of the area about the dog control programme and solicit the support of all the residents reassuring them that the local authority is taking adequate steps for their safety.
6. The captured dogs shall be brought to the dog kennels/dog pounds managed by the animal welfare organisations. On reaching the dog pounds, all the dogs shall be examined by the veterinarians and healthy and sick dogs should be segregated. Sick dogs should be given proper treatment in the hospitals run by the SPCA/other recognised institutions, and only after they are treated, they should be sterilised and vaccinated. The dogs will be sterilised/vaccinated under the supervision of the veterinarians of the hospital run by the SPCA, animal welfare organisation, or other dog shelters. After necessary period of follow-up, the dogs shall be released at the same place or locality from where they were captured, and the date, time, and place of their release shall be recorded. The representative of animal welfare organisations shall accompany the dog squad at the time of release also.
7. At a time only one lot of dogs shall be brought for sterilisation and immunisation at one dog kennel or dog pound, and these dogs shall be from one locality. Two lots from different

areas or localities shall not be mixed at the same dog pound or dog kennel.

8. The dog kennel must have sufficient space for proper housing and free movement of dogs. The place should have proper ventilation and natural lighting and must be kept clean. Adults and puppies must be housed separately, and among the adults, the males and females also should be housed separately. Adequate arrangement for drinking water and food shall be made for dogs while in captivity.
9. Female dogs found to be pregnant shall not undergo abortion (irrespective of stage of pregnancy) and sterilisation and should be released till they have litter.

7.2.5.6 Identification and Recording

ABC Rules prescribe that sterilised dogs shall be vaccinated before release and the ears of these dogs should be either clipped and/or tattooed for being identified as sterilised or immunised dogs. In addition, the dogs may be given token or nylon collars for identification and detailed records of such dogs shall be maintained. Branding of dogs would not be permitted.

7.2.5.7 Euthanasia of Street Dogs

ABC Rules have a provision that incurably ill and mortally wounded dogs as diagnosed by a qualified veterinarian appointed by the committee shall be euthanised during specified hours in a humane manner by administering sodium pentothal for adult dogs and thiopental intraperitoneal for puppies by a qualified veterinarian or euthanised in any other humane manner approved by AWBI. No dog shall be euthanised in the presence of another dog. The person responsible for euthanising shall make sure that the animal is dead, before disposal.

7.2.5.8 Furious or Dumb Rabid Dogs

1. On receipt of complaints from the public to the Dog Control Cell of the local authority, or on its own, the dog squad of the local authority would catch such dogs, suspected to be rabid.
2. The caught dog would then be taken to the pound where it would be isolated in an isolation ward.
3. The suspected rabid dog would then be subjected to inspection by a panel of two persons, i.e. a veterinary surgeon appointed by the local authority and a representative from an animal welfare organisation.
4. If the dog is found to have a high probability of having rabies, it would be isolated till it dies a natural death. Death normally occurs within 10 days of contracting rabies. Premature killing of suspected rabid dogs, therefore, prevents the true incidence of rabies from being known and appropriate action being taken.
5. If the dog is found not to have rabies but some other disease, it would be handed over to the animal welfare organisations who will take necessary action to cure and rehabilitate the dog.

7.2.5.9 Disposal of Carcasses

The carcasses of such euthanised dogs shall be disposed of in an incinerator to be provided by the local authority.

7.2.5.10 Guidelines for Breeders

1. A breeder must be registered with AWBI.
2. Breeders must maintain full record of the number of puppies born/died from individual bitches.
3. A breeder must maintain record of the person buying the puppies. He should ensure that the buyer has the required knowledge for the upkeep of the puppies.

7.2.5.11 Application of Rules Where Local Bye-laws Exist

If there is in force in any area to which the ABC Rules extend, any Act, rule, regulation, or bye-law made under any law for the time being in force by the state or the local authority in respect of any of the matters for which provision is made in the ABC rules, such rule, regulation, or bye-law shall to the extent to which:

(a) It contains provisions less irksome to the animal than those contained in these rules, shall prevail
(b) It contains provisions more irksome to the animal than those contained in ABC Rules, be of no effect

7.2.6 Animal Birth Control (ABC) Programme in India

AWBI is promoting the implementation of ABC-AR Programme in almost all major cities of India. Over 100,000 stray dogs are sterilised and vaccinated against rabies every year under the ABC Rules. The ABC Programme has been operating in over 60 cities all over India, including Delhi, Jaipur, Chennai, Mumbai, Bangalore, Hyderabad, Kolkata, Jodhpur, and Kalimpong. In Tamil Nadu and Goa, the ABC-AR Programme has been successfully implemented for the entire state since 2007. This has led to Tamil Nadu state pioneering a new concept of a Participatory Model of the ABC Programme in 50 Municipalities and 5 Municipal Corporations, with 50 % cost sharing by local bodies on participatory basis. Delhi has adopted the Participatory Model of the ABC Programme since 2008 (AWBI 2009).

7.2.6.1 Standard Operating Procedures for ABC Programme in India

AWBI has brought out the Standard Operating Procedures (SOP) manual (AWBI 2009) to carry out ABC projects for effective population control of street/stray dogs with a uniform and standard code of professional practice, efficiently, diligently, and humanely. This SOP manual provides detailed guidelines on all aspects of the ABC Programme including techniques for humane catching and transportation of stray dogs, identification methods, record keeping, basic infrastructure requirements, anaesthetic and surgical protocols, and preoperative and post-operative care. It also includes the guidelines for humane euthanasia of dogs and safe disposal of carcasses. It is mandatory for all animal welfare organisations implementing the ABC programme in the country to follow these guidelines.

7.3 Canine Rabies Control

Though human fatality due to rabies can be substantially reduced by the application of protective vaccines and RIG, it is difficult to attain true success in rabies control without controlling and eliminating the disease at the source, mainly dogs, which constitute the largest single source of rabies exposures resulting in human deaths. Canine rabies control programmes reduce the disease not only in canines but eventually result in decline in the human rabies incidence too at a much lower cost. This is so because human rabies biologicals are usually much more expensive than animal vaccines. Effective canine rabies vaccination is thus an indispensable component of any rabies control programme.

Many developed nations have successfully controlled rabies in animals. For example, the United States (USA) annually spends US$ over 300 million for rabies prevention, most of which is spent on dog vaccinations. Due to an annual turnover of approximately 25 % in the dog population, revaccination of millions of animals is required each year. Rabies control programmes require continuous operation to prevent reintroduction of rabies in an area from the infected animals coming from other areas (CDC 2012).

Modern veterinary vaccines are now widely available and affordable in the developing countries. These are highly immunogenic inactivated cell culture vaccines for immunisation of dogs via the parenteral route. For mass canine vaccination, use of inactivated rabies vaccine is recommended over live vaccine because the management of inactivated vaccine in the field is easier and it is less sensitive to changes in temperature. Further, inactivated vaccines do not cause any risk to the vaccinator due to accidental self-inoculation. There is increasing use of these for animal immunisation due to recent improvements in vaccine production techniques (WHO 2012b). Combined vaccines including rabies vaccine and vaccines against other diseases are also available for dogs and cats.

For a successful vaccination campaign, vaccination of dogs should be done in a planned, organised way. At least 75 % of the dog population in each community should be vaccinated within a month. In areas where the dog population turnover is rapid, it may be necessary to carry out a mass vaccination campaign each year (Figs. 7.5 and 7.6). However, if the vaccine produces effective immunity for longer period and the system for

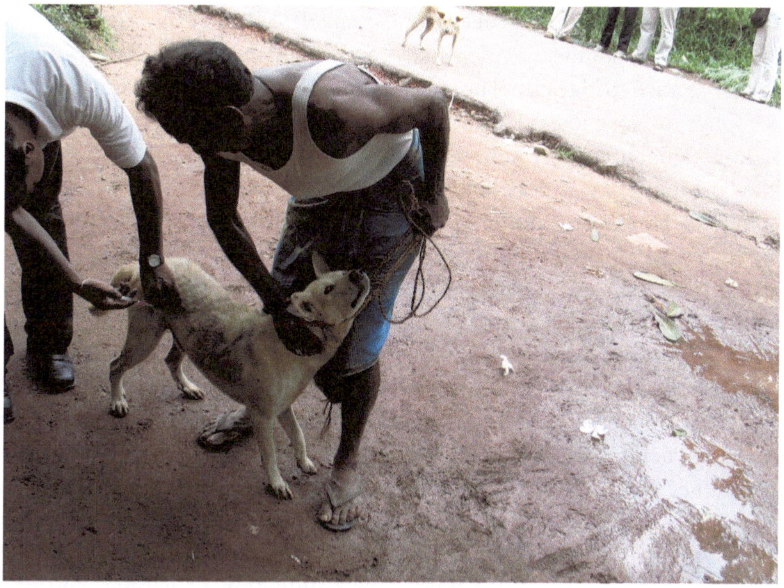

Fig. 7.5 Stray dog vaccination (Photo courtesy: Dr. Deborrah Briggs)

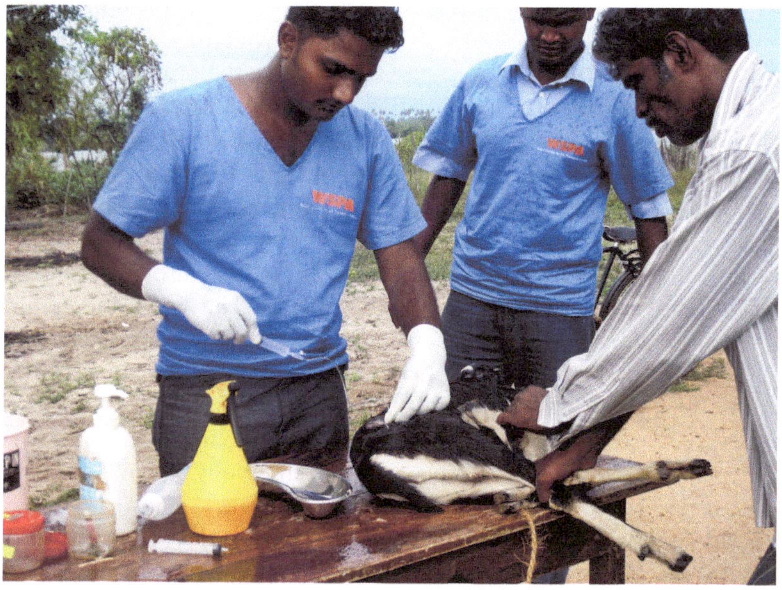

Fig. 7.6 Rabies vaccination in Sri Lanka after tsunami (Photo credit: WSPA)

identifying vaccinated dogs can be trusted to last more than 1 year, the advantage of longer immunity may be taken by vaccinating only the dogs entering the population after the last campaign. Revaccination of dogs covered during the last campaign can then be done at intervals of about 2 years (WHO 2012b).

Full implementation of dog vaccination programmes may be expensive. For example, the cost of dog vaccination typically ranges between US$1.19 and US$4.27 per dog vaccinated in a range of rural and urban settings when a central-point vaccination strategy is adopted, which is the most cost-effective strategy. This includes consumable costs (vaccine, syringes, needles, certificates, registers, collars, stationery), delivery (staff costs, transport), storage (fridges, cool boxes), and societal costs (days of work lost). The house-to-house vaccination campaigns tend to be more expensive and the cost may vary widely between different communities. However, adopting this strategy may be necessary in some situations to reach sufficient vaccination coverage (Partners for Rabies Prevention 2010). The cost can be reduced through involvement of volunteers in the vaccination campaigns, through careful consideration of logistics and transport costs, and by holding well-planned synchronised campaigns.

The task of dog rabies control in India is really enormous due to large dog population. It is, therefore, essential to chalk out programmes for dog population management besides innovating cost-effective animal vaccine delivery systems in the country.

7.4 Wildlife Rabies Control

Some countries have been successful in controlling rabies in dogs by implementing vigilant control measures, but with the decline in dog rabies, the role of sylvatic or wildlife rabies has come to the fore. Today, in European countries and the USA, more rabies cases are reported in wild animals than in domestic animals, and a considerable proportion of both human and domestic animal exposures to the disease are the result of wild animal contact.

Rabies in Europe is predominately sylvatic rabies, with wildlife species accounting for approximately 80 % of all rabies cases. Of these, more than 80 % are red foxes (*Vulpes vulpes*) (Rabies Bulletin Europe 2012). In the USA, 92 % of reported cases of rabies in the year 2010 were due to wild animals, mainly raccoons, skunks, bats, foxes, and other including rodents and lagomorphs. Outbreaks of rabies infections in raccoons, skunks, foxes, and coyotes are found in broad geographical regions across the country (CDC 2012).

The emergence of wildlife as principal rabies vector has added a complex dimension to rabies control. While dog rabies can be effectively controlled through different simple strategies, the same kind of measures may not be directly applicable to wildlife (Hanlon et al. 1999).

7.4.1 Methods of Control

General approaches to controlling rabies in wildlife include reduction or elimination of the reservoir species and elimination of rabies in the reservoir species (Figs. 7.7, 7.8 and 7.9). Another option includes protection of the victim species from the reservoir species. It involves reducing the opportunities of interaction or contact of wildlife with humans, pets, or livestock by certain measures, such as garbage management, modification or elimination of habitat, and proper storage or removal of human and pet foods (Hanlon et al. 1999; Rupprecht et al. 2001; Rosatte 2011). These methods may be applied in combination.

Initially, culling and destruction of reservoir species was the primary rabies control measure, but during the past few decades, there have been significant changes in the tactics of wildlife rabies control. The advances in the research and development of oral rabies vaccines and delivery systems for wildlife have now made it feasible to apply the control measures to substantially large areas. This has led to elimination of rabies from many territories (Rosatte 2011). Hanlon et al. (1999) and Rosatte (2011) have published detailed descriptions of the historical and contemporary methods of rabies control in wildlife. These are briefly summarised below.

7.4.1.1 Rabies Vector Population Reduction

The conventional method of population control aims at reducing the densities of rabies vector species resulting in disruption of the natural route of spread of infection among the animal population. For this, a number of techniques such as trapping and euthanasia, hunting, poison baits, and gassing have been used. However, such programmes are generally quite labour-intensive, cost prohibitive, and ecologically and ethically unacceptable (Hanlon et al. 1999; Rupprecht

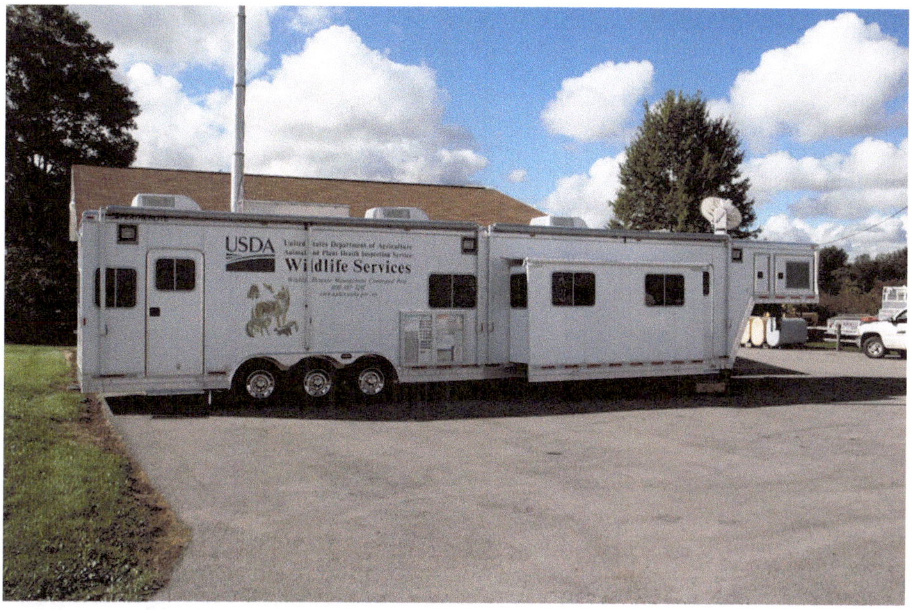

Fig. 7.7 USDA-APHIS Wildlife Services (Photo credit: USDA-APHIS)

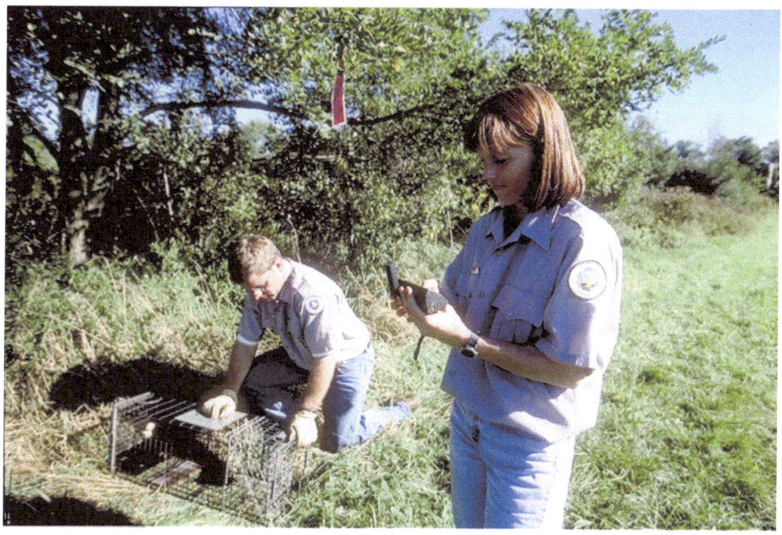

Fig. 7.8 Wildlife rabies management (Photo credit: USDA-APHIS)

et al. 2001; Rosatte 2011). Moreover, it has been observed that these methods alone are incapable of reducing and maintaining the vector population below a certain threshold level and it may not be possible to decrease the rabies incidence effectively (Rabies Bulletin Europe 2012). Due to the impracticability, this approach has limited utility in large-scale application.

7.4.1.2 Fertility Control

Research has been done to lower the fertility of animals through reproductive inhibitors, thus controlling the rabies vector population growth. However, this method has not been very successful because of lack of safe, effective, and long-lasting agents and effective delivery systems (Hanlon et al. 1999; Rosatte 2011).

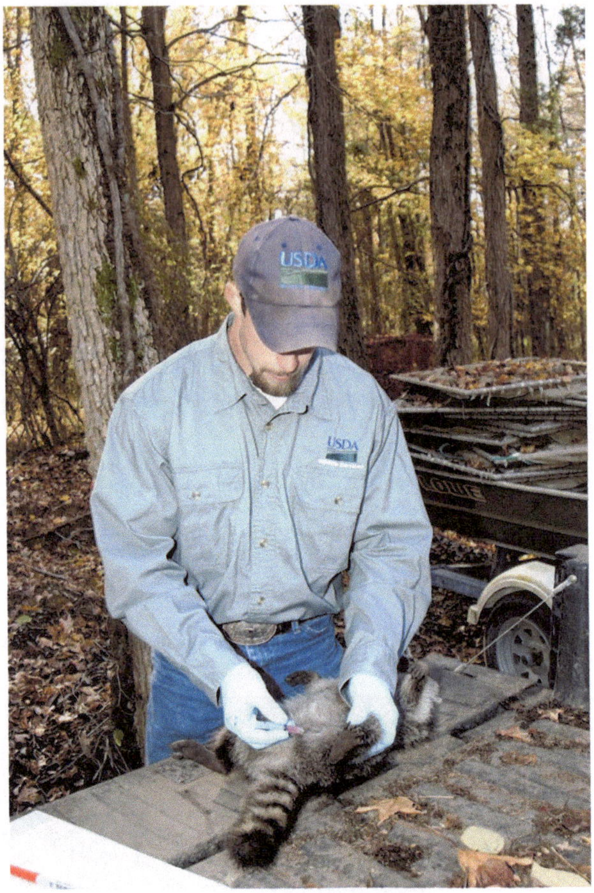

Fig. 7.9 Wildlife rabies management. Collection of tissue sample from an anesthetised raccoon to determine the protective status of oral vaccination (Photo credit: USDA-APHIS)

7.4.1.3 Habitat Modification

Habitat modification is aimed at reducing the chance of interaction of potential rabies vectors like skunks, raccoons, and bats with human beings, pets, and livestock. It can be achieved by using animal-proof garbage containers or enclosures, frequent garbage disposal, making pet food inaccessible to wild animals, capping chimneys, and screening louvre vents. Similarly, techniques may be improvised to prevent access of bats to human habitations (Hanlon et al. 1999).

7.4.1.4 Trap–Vaccinate–Release Programmes

Vaccination of reservoir species has been shown to be more effective and economically beneficial than the wildlife population control approach. Trap–vaccinate–release (TVR) approach is one of the two potential methods of vaccinating wildlife reservoir species, the other being oral rabies vaccination. In TVR approach, targeted reservoir species are livetrapped and manually injected with liquid vaccine. The difficulty faced in capturing of wild animals and administration of parenteral vaccine reduces the feasibility of TVR programmes (Hanlon et al. 1999; Rosatte 2011).

7.4.1.5 Oral Rabies Vaccination

Oral rabies vaccination (ORV) has been found to be a very cost-effective method and has been extremely successful in red foxes and raccoon dogs in Europe. It involves vaccinating the animals through baits containing oral vaccine. The ORV is practically a very feasible approach that can be applied on a very large scale to increase herd immunity even in the cases where the probability of trapping the wildlife vectors is low. Contemporary advances in the research and development of oral rabies vaccines and delivery systems have now made it feasible to distribute millions of vaccine baits over thousands of square kilometres of habitat to control rabies in wildlife rabies vectors (Rosatte 2011).

7.5 Oral Rabies Vaccination in Animals

ORV represents a socially acceptable methodology that may be applied on a broad geographical scale to manage the disease in specific terrestrial wildlife reservoirs. It has proven its utility as a cost-effective tactic and has been extremely successful in Europe in controlling rabies in red foxes and raccoon dogs (*Nyctereutes procyonoides*), and many countries have attained "rabies-free" status (Rosatte 2011). The application of ORV has also shown promising results in controlling rabies in foxes in Canada and in coyotes and grey foxes in the USA (Rosatte 2011). The feasibility of application of ORV in stray dogs has also been demonstrated in some countries.

Oral vaccines are distributed in baits over a large area; hence the safety aspects of the vaccine baits released into the environment would require utmost attention. The WHO (2012b) recommends the assessment of the safety of a candidate vaccine for the target and nontarget species as given below:

- The candidate vaccine strain should be characterised according to procedures recommended for rabies vaccines for veterinary use.
- The vaccine chosen should not produce any disease in 10 young (3–6 months old) animals belonging to the target species when administered orally at 10 times the dose recommended for field use.
- The possibility of excretion of vaccine virus in the saliva of the animals should also be examined. Following immunisation, swabs should be taken daily. No virus should be present after 3–4 days. Any virus recovered should be characterised using MAb.
- Where feasible, at least 10 and if possibly 50 of each of the most common local rodent species should be given the field dose of vaccine (i.e. the dose which is contained in a bait) orally and intramuscularly. No more than 10 % of the animals so vaccinated should exhibit sickness or mortality due to rabies.
- Relevant local wild or domestic animal species that may take baits should be examined using MAb to ensure that no vaccine-induced rabies has occurred (WHO 2012b).

The development of recombinant DNA technology has initiated a new era in rabies control. Recombinant vaccines cannot exhibit residual pathogenicity caused by rabies because they contain only single non-virulent gene products. The majority of the safety requirements for modified live-virus vaccines are also applicable to recombinant vaccines (WHO 2012b).

7.5.1 Application of ORV in Wildlife

The first field trial on ORV of foxes was successfully conducted in Switzerland in 1978. Chicken-head baits containing SAD-Berne ORV were used. Between October 1978 and October 1990, 1.3 million such baits were distributed in the country. Continual surveillance led to detection of three cases of vaccine-induced rabies. No other vaccine-related deaths were noted in over 900 animals examined. Baits containing SAD-B19 vaccine were also used in Europe to control fox rabies. Since 1983, millions of baits containing this virus have been distributed in Europe, including Belgium, France, Germany, Italy, Luxembourg, and a number of Eastern European countries with no reported deaths among nontarget species. Other vaccine strains (SAG 1, SAG 2, ERA, Vnukovo-32) have been distributed in certain Western European countries, Canada, and the Russian Federation (Rosatte 2011; WHO 2012b).

The application of ORV for rabies control in terrestrial vectors (red foxes and raccoon dogs) showed excellent results in Europe as the annual number of rabies cases in Europe dropped from 21,000 in the year 1990 to 5,400 in 2004. Rabies has been successfully controlled and eradicated in most parts of Western and Central Europe. So far several countries including Finland, the Netherlands (1991), Italy (1997), Switzerland (1998), France (2000), Belgium, Luxembourg

(2001), Czech Republic (2004), Germany (2008), and Austria (2008) have been declared as being officially free of terrestrial rabies. In 2009, Italy was reinfected by fox rabies, and ORV is currently applied as a control measure (Rosatte 2011; Rabies Bulletin Europe 2012).

In North America, ORV has been under field investigation since 1985 in Canada and since 1990 in the USA. Raboral V-RG® is currently the only effective oral vaccine licensed for use in free-ranging raccoons, grey foxes, and coyotes in the USA. In the year 2007 alone, more than 12 million vaccine baits were distributed over 241,350 km^2 area in the country. The figures for the years 2005 and 2006 were also almost similar. In all, there have been nearly 48 million doses of the vaccine distributed in the USA and Canada, and 63 million doses have been dispersed worldwide (USDA 2012).

7.5.1.1 Vaccine Delivery Systems

ORV utilises baits attractive to targeted reservoir species. When the bait is taken (bitten) by the animal, it releases an encapsulated, attenuated rabies virus vaccine into the mouth or pharyngeal tissues of the animal to elicit an immune response. During the first field trial of ORV in the late 1970s, chicken heads were used as bait, to which SAD-Bern vaccine in plastic capsule was stapled. Nowadays, usually a vaccine-filled sachet is enveloped by a bait casing typically consisting of fishmeal, fat, and paraffin (Figs. 7.10 and 7.11).

Raboral V-RG consists of a plastic sachet containing the vaccine (about 1.5 ml) which is enclosed in solid fishmeal polymer bait or is coated with wax and fishmeal crumbs. In the USA, the outer bait matrix is made from fishmeal (for raccoons and coyotes) or dog food (for grey foxes) combined with a polymer that acts as a binding agent. The sachet inside the bait matrix is waxed into place so that it does not fall out during aerial delivery. As the raccoon, grey fox, or coyote eats through the outer bait matrix, the inner sachet gets punctured and the vaccine enters the animal's mouth and coats the lymphatic tissue in the throat, eliciting immune response (USDA 2012). Similarly, ONRAB vaccine is contained in bait consisting of a plastic blister pack surrounded by a wax- and fat-based matrix containing tetracycline hydrochloride marker.

Vaccine baits need to be deposited throughout all potential habitats of the vector animal which is usually a very large area. Different vaccine bait distribution systems have been developed. Aerial distribution preferably by aircraft or by helicopter is the most efficient way (Fig. 7.12). Aerial distribution is generally done in rural areas. The bait distribution machine is controlled from the airplane and is turned off when crossing a road or house to avoid human contact with the bait. Baiting by hand (Fig. 7.13) is done in urban and suburban areas to increase the chances of uptake of the bait by the target species while minimising the chances of human contact with the bait (Rabies Bulletin Europe 2012; USDA 2012).

7.5.2 Application of ORV in Stray Dogs

The programmes of mass vaccination of dogs by parenteral route in developing countries often face hurdles due to the resource crunch for handling a large number of stray dogs. Oral vaccines allow for easy mass vaccination and offer new approaches promising a significant increase in the dog vaccination coverage (especially of free-roaming and poorly supervised dogs), both when applied exclusively or in combination with parenteral vaccination (WHO 2007). However, since dogs, unlike wild animals, live in close vicinity of human habitations, there is likelihood of exposure of human beings to the vaccine baits during ORV programmes for dogs. The candidate vaccines thus have to meet certain requirements regarding safety for the nontarget species, particularly human beings. Further, it has to be ensured that the vaccines are efficacious and cost-effective.

The WHO has published recommendations concerning evaluation of safety and efficacy of ORV for application in dogs (WHO 2007). Several pilot studies conducted in different countries including Sri Lanka, the Philippines, India, and China have shown the feasibility, efficacy, and safety of ORV in dogs (Perera et al. 2000;

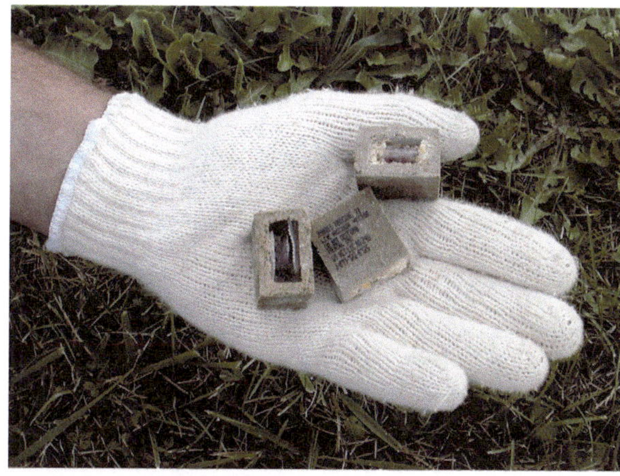

Fig. 7.10 Oral rabies vaccine in fishmeal polymer bait (Photo credit: USDA-APHIS)

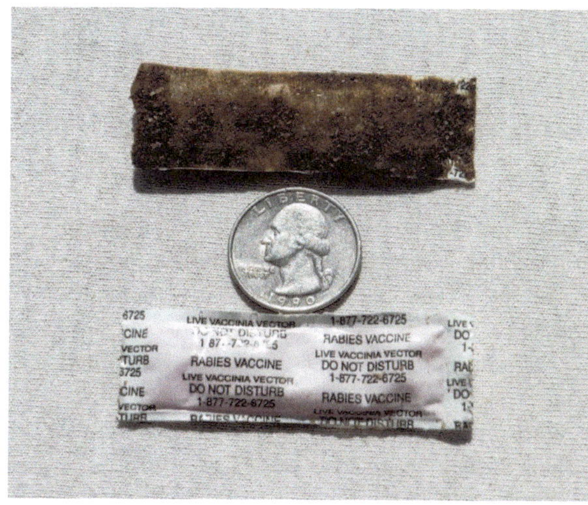

Fig. 7.11 Oral rabies vaccine in coated sachet bait (Photo credit: USDA-APHIS)

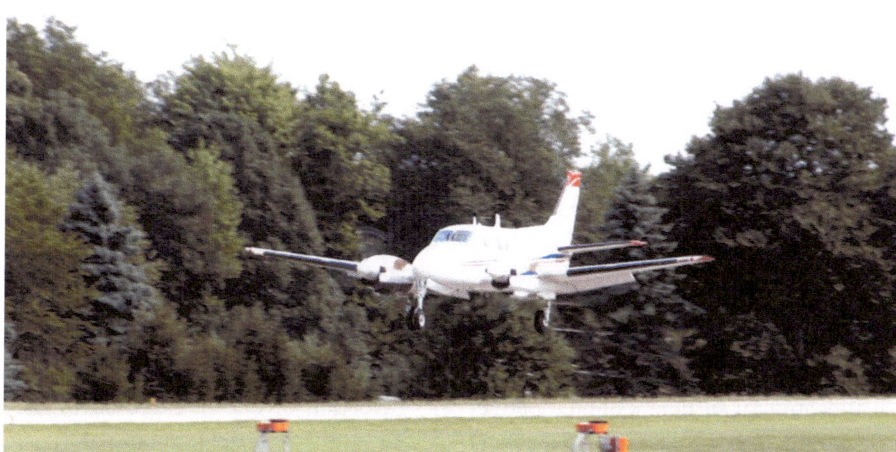

Fig. 7.12 Aircraft facility for oral rabies vaccine bait distribution (Photo credit: USDA-APHIS)

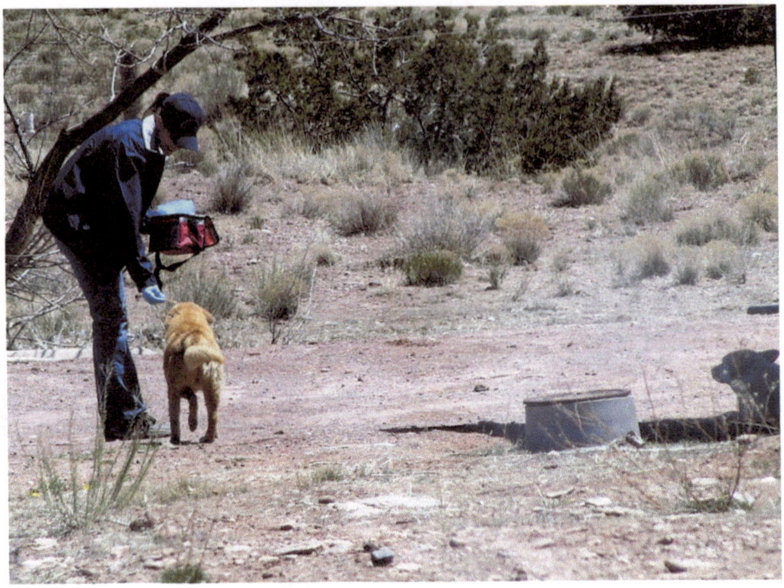

Fig. 7.13 Oral rabies vaccination by hand baiting (Photo credit: USDA-APHIS)

Estrada et al. 2001; Cliquet et al. 2007; Zhang et al. 2008). However, elaborate studies may be necessary before the technique is practically adopted.

According to the WHO (2007), the individual countries should study the opportunity of introducing oral vaccination in their rabies control strategy. The countries should examine the potential role of oral vaccination of dogs and should consider applying it only after the traditional control measures, such as establishing or strengthening the surveillance of rabies and vaccinating dogs by the parenteral route, have yielded less than optimal results from the epidemiological and economical points of view. The following qualification criteria (WHO 2007) should be considered when a country contemplates the use of oral vaccination of dogs:

- Dog rabies is endemic.
- A dog rabies vaccination programme by parenteral vaccination is in place for the last 5 years and is properly monitored and evaluated.
- There is allocation of sufficient annual budget for the operation of the rabies surveillance and control programme.
- There is a network of biomedical services and diagnostic laboratories with the facility of standard immunofluorescent techniques in the country.
- The data on human and animal rabies cases are available for at least 5 previous years.
- The information on dog demography including dog population size estimates, density, distribution, age structure, and turnover is available.

Further, when pilot research projects using oral rabies vaccines in dogs are considered, a national team should be constituted that includes specialists of dog ecology. The WHO staff and/or staff from relevant WHO Collaborating Centres should be closely associated with the programme. The team leader should establish the working plan for oral vaccination projects. The population or subpopulation of dogs intended for oral vaccination should be identified and a strategy to reach these animals should be elaborated. The WHO (2007) recommends the following initial steps for the programme:

- Selection of one or more candidate vaccines that fulfil the safety and efficacy requirements described by the WHO (2007)

- Determination of vaccine efficacy in local captive dogs by oral administration
- Evaluation of vaccine in terms of national requirements regarding the introduction into the country, even for experimental purpose
- Testing of vaccine safety on major local nontarget species competitors for baits which have not already been tested for safety with the selected vaccine(s)
- Selection of bait out of the available options or to developing a new bait according to local conditions
- Selection or evolving methods of bait delivery according to the population or subpopulation of dogs which are targeted
- Evaluation of the possibility, extent, and circumstances of human exposure to the vaccine/bait through placebo trials
- Evaluation of the acceptability of the selected bait in the target population through placebo baiting trials
- Providing sufficient information to the public before undertaking any field trial to elicit general public support and cooperation

According to the recommendations, a total population vaccination level of 80 % is desired. Repeat vaccination campaigns should be conducted when population vaccination levels drop below 60 %. Adequate long-lasting marking of dogs is important for evaluation of vaccination coverage (WHO 2007).

7.6 Success Stories in Rabies Control

Despite all odds, marked success in rabies control has been demonstrated in many parts of the world during the past three decades. As a result, not only has rabies declined in dogs and other animals, but human rabies deaths have also been substantially reduced or eliminated. Such highly successful programmes have been carried out in many countries including developing countries in Asia and South America. A brief description of some successful programmes given below demonstrates that it is feasible to control and even eliminate canine rabies and prevent human rabies deaths with systematic concerted efforts.

7.6.1 Success in Europe

The stepwise intensive efforts to control and eliminate both canine and wildlife-mediated rabies have shown unprecedented results in the European countries. Large parts of Western, Northern, and Central Europe are officially recognised as free from terrestrial rabies. In Western Europe, currently all measures are directed towards the maintenance of a rabies-free status by avoiding reintroduction of the disease including implementation of the pet travel scheme, risk-based surveillance, and establishment of cordon sanitaire along borders to rabies-endemic regions (Müller and Freuling 2011).

7.6.2 Success in Latin America

The elimination of human rabies transmitted by dogs in the Region of the Americas by 2005 was a decision made by all Pan American Health Organization (PAHO) member states in the 1980s. Since then, these countries have made major efforts to eliminate rabies with marked success and the Region is very close to reaching its goal of eliminating dog-transmitted human rabies. Part of Latin America has already managed to eliminate the spread of the rabies virus in the canine population. A large part of the Southern Cone – Chile and Uruguay, vast areas of Argentina, and all of Southern Brazil, including São Paulo and Rio de Janeiro – is already free of dog rabies. Panama and Costa Rica are in a similar situation, as are some departments of Peru (PAHO 2012). However, recently in December 2011, after 30 years with no detected cases of terrestrial animal rabies, a cat with rabies virus was diagnosed and confirmed in São Paulo state in Brazil (Taylor and Romijn 2012). The cat was not vaccinated as the government of São Paulo had decided to suspend the free rabies vaccination programme for pets in 2010, following several adverse reactions to a rabies vaccine administered to dogs and cats (including some fatalities). The cat was probably infected by a bat because cats may chase a rabies-infected bat which is unable to fly and may be bitten by the bat in the process. Because the disease had been virtually eliminated from São Paulo state by vaccination, this case is particularly alarming. The Ministry of Health had recently suspended vaccination of pets in 15 Brazilian states, which have also not recorded the occurrences of rabies cases in recent years, but it has now decided to restart vaccination campaigns across the whole country (Taylor and Romijn 2012).

Analysis of the trend in rabies cases in Latin America during the period 1982–2003 reveals 91 % decline in the number of human cases from 355 to 35. Rabies in dogs declined by 93 % from 15,686 cases to 1131 during this period. From 1990 to 2003, dogs were the source of infection in 65 % of reported human cases, which fell from 152 to 27 (Schneider et al. 2005; Belotto et al. 2005; PAHO 2012). By the year 2010, 95 % reduction in the cases of human and canine rabies was achieved. Approximately 350 human cases and 3,000 canine in the early 1980s were reduced to less than 10 and 100 cases, respectively, in 2010 (Tamayo et al. 2011). This sharp reduction is attributable mainly to the control measures implemented by the countries of the Region, such as the mass vaccination of dogs and prophylactic treatment for people who have been exposed. In Latin America, about 44 million dogs are vaccinated every year, and approximately one million people at risk of contracting the disease are tended to, 25 % of them receiving postexposure treatment. More than 100 national and regional laboratories are engaged in rabies diagnosis and have processed nearly 74,000 samples per year indicating the extent of efforts being made towards achieving the target of rabies elimination (Schneider et al. 2005; Belotto et al. 2005; PAHO 2012).

Among the Latin American countries, Mexico has shown particularly remarkable success. National Rabies Control Programme using mass parenteral vaccination of dogs in the country started in 1990 and about seven million dogs were vaccinated the same year. The number of vaccinated dogs exceeded 10 and 15 million in 1995 and 2005, respectively. Between 1990 and 2005, more than 150 million vaccine doses of modern cell culture-based inactivated rabies virus vaccines were administered. As a result, human cases due to dog-mediated rabies decreased from 60 in 1990 to 0 in 2000. The number of rabies cases in dogs decreased from 3,049 in 1990 to 70 (Lucas et al. 2008).

7.6.3 Success in the USA

Over the past 100 years, the scenario of rabies in the USA has changed dramatically. Animal control and vaccination programmes started in the 1940s and ORV programmes in the 2000s have eliminated the role of domestic dogs as reservoirs of rabies in the country. Consequently, now more than 90 % of all animal cases reported annually to the CDC occur in wildlife while before 1960 the majority was in domestic animals (CDC 2012).

The number of rabies-related human deaths in the USA has declined from more than 100 annually at the turn of the twentieth century to one or two per year in the 1990s. Apart from dog rabies control, the use of effective human rabies vaccines and immunoglobulin has made it possible. In the USA, human fatalities associated with rabies occur in people who fail to seek medical assistance, usually because they were unaware of their exposure (CDC 2012).

7.6.4 Success in Sri Lanka

Sri Lanka has registered a sharp decline in the number of human rabies deaths through mass dog vaccination campaigns, improved accessibility to human PEP, and an effective vaccine delivery system. Mass vaccination of dogs has shown great impact on human rabies cases in the country. The number of dogs that were vaccinated each year was increased rapidly from few thousand in the year 1975 to more than 800,000 in 2005 and 1,000,000 in 2008. With the result, the human rabies incidence per 1,000,000 persons, which was more than 2 in the year 1975, declined to less than 1 in 1985 and less than 0.5 in the year 2005 onwards. The country has adopted cost-effective intradermal rabies vaccination to control human rabies (WHO 2008).

7.6.5 Success in KwaZulu-Natal (South Africa)

With international cooperation between the WHO, the Bill and Melinda Gates Foundation, the South African authorities, and other rabies experts, a pilot canine rabies elimination programme was started in 2009 in KwaZulu-Natal, a province in South Africa. In 2011, KwaZulu-Natal was able to declare no recorded human deaths from rabies in a 1-year period for the first time in over 20 years. Extensive training of health professionals and public awareness together with the motivation provided by international attention have been major factors in the project's success (Rabiesblueprint 2012). The 5-year project aims to achieve elimination of human and dog rabies from KwaZulu-Natal by 2014 (WHO 2012b).

7.6.6 Success in Bohol (Philippines)

The Philippines is among the top 10 countries facing rabies deaths. In 2007, when the Global Alliance for Rabies Control (GARC) began the Bohol Rabies Prevention and Elimination Project, Bohol Island was ranked as the 4th highest rabies-affected region in the Philippines, averaging 10 deaths per year. In 2010, that number was zero. Though there has been one death in 2011, the project has caused tremendous improvement (GARC 2012b). This programme produced a seismic shift in rabies control in Bohol by turning it from the government-dependent implementation to a community-led movement involving thousands of village-based volunteers and teachers apart from some paid government staff. The project has received the prestigious Galing Pook award from the President of the Philippines for its excellence.

The programme steadily enforced mandatory dog registration and vaccination and used the registration fee collections to fund the ongoing programme costs and to subsidise human postexposure vaccines. Now, almost all dogs are registered and have dog tags. Seventy percent of the dog population has been vaccinated and registered, involving 47 municipalities, 109 villages, and 43,690 households. The project envisages inclusion of rabies education in the primary school curriculum and teaching over 185,000 children every year about rabies, bite prevention, and responsible pet ownership in schools.

Besides saving lives, the project has helped tourism industry flourish, contributing to the local economy. An unexpected benefit of the project includes a significant reduction in the number of road accidents caused by stray dogs. The project itself is expanding and it has plans to use the rabies control infrastructure for simultaneously controlling other diseases.

7.6.7 Afya Serengeti Rabies Control Project

The Serengeti region is a sprawling and diverse stretch of land located in Tanzania in the eastern part of Africa. At the centre of the region is the Serengeti National Park, a controlled-access, protected wildlife conservation area bordered by multiple districts containing many small villages that are the focus of the Afya Serengeti project. Started as a research project in 1997, it is now a rabies control project that works with local people in the Serengeti to ensure widespread vaccination of domestic dogs (Afya 2012).

The project's successes include reduction of hospitalisations due to rabid dog bites by 92 %, elimination of rabies from the Serengeti National Park itself and the adjacent Ngorongoro District, and no reported rabies outbreaks in areas where a 70 % vaccination rate has been achieved. The vaccination has also helped in protection of African wild dogs that were threatened with extinction due to outbreaks of rabies in 1990. As a result of the operation of the project, there is increase in the population of African wild dogs in and around the park by 17 % each year (Afya 2012). Because of the remarkable success of vaccination efforts in the Serengeti, plans are also underway to expand the project into other countries.

7.7 Coordinated Efforts Against Rabies

A number of rabies surveillance and control programmes have demonstrated that human exposure to rabies can be substantially reduced by controlling and eliminating rabies in dog populations and wildlife vectors. Though mass vaccination of dogs is the single most cost-effective method to control and eliminate dog rabies, the other interventions such as animal birth control, promotion of responsible dog ownership, compulsory notification of rabies in humans and animals, ensuring the availability of reliable diagnostic procedures, and confirmation of cases of rabies are also important (WHO 2010). It all involves multisector coordination.

7.7.1 WHO Initiatives

The WHO promotes widespread initiatives not only in the direction of prevention of rabies through PEP in human beings but also for control and elimination of canine rabies (WHO 2012b). The major activities of WHO in these directions are listed below:

- Promoting wider access to postexposure treatment with modern vaccines
- Promoting the use of the multisite intradermal regimen to reduce the cost of postexposure treatments
- Promoting domestic production of rabies biologicals
- Promoting consistent availability of modern rabies vaccines for humans and for animals
- Improving rabies surveillance
- Developing documents and guidelines for comprehensive rabies control programmes
- Implementation of canine rabies control and elimination programmes
- Organisation of sustainable mass dog vaccination campaigns
- Stimulation of studies on oral vaccination of dogs and development of safer and effective oral vaccines and baits
- Implementation of dog population management programmes
- Continuing education of health and veterinary professionals in rabies prevention and control
- Increasing awareness in the public and in the medical profession about rabies prevention and prevention
- Eliciting political support for rabies control programmes

The WHO has a worldwide rabies network. It is working together with numerous collaborating centres and other organisations to reduce the impact of rabies worldwide, with the overall goal of human rabies eradication (Rabies Bulletin Europe 2012). The list of WHO Collaborating Centres for Rabies Research (updated to July 2012) is given in Box 7.2.

7.7.2 OIE Initiatives

The World Organisation for Animal Health (OIE) is committed to the cause of worldwide eradication of rabies. It maintains a dedicated rabies web portal and provides science-based standards, guidelines, and recommendations for the control of rabies in animals and to prevent its spread through trade. It also provides standards for the diagnosis of the disease and the preparation of vaccines for use in animals.

The OIE has a network of OIE Reference Laboratories designated for rabies. These function as centres of expertise and standardisation of diagnostic techniques. Leading and active researchers are functioning as the Reference Experts in these laboratories. They provide scientific and technical assistance and expert advice on surveillance and control of the disease. They also provide scientific and technical training for member countries and territories and coordinate scientific and technical studies in collaboration with other laboratories or organisations. Through this network of Reference Laboratories and Collaborating Centres, the OIE provides policy advice, strategy design, and technical assistance for the diagnosis, control, and eradication of rabies (OIE 2013). The list of Reference Experts and Laboratories on Rabies (updated to June 2013) is given in Box 7.3.

Box 7.2 WHO Collaborating Centres for Rabies Research (Rabies Bulletin Europe 2012)

1. WHO Collaborating Centre for Control, Pathogenesis and Epidemiology of Rabies in Carnivores, Centre of Expertise (COFE) for Rabies, Ottawa Laboratory Fallowfield (OLF), Canadian Food Inspection Agency, Nepean (Ontario), Canada
2. WHO Collaborating Centre for Reference and Research on Rabies, Rabies Section, Division of Viral & Rickettsial Diseases (DVRD), Viral and Rickettsial Zoonoses Branch, National Center for Infectious Diseases (NCID), Centers for Disease Control & Prevention (CDC), Atlanta, USA
3. WHO Collaborating Centre for Reference & Research on Rabies, The Wistar Institute, Philadelphia, USA
4. WHO Collaborating Centre for Reference and Research on Rabies, Unité de la Rage, Institut Pasteur, Paris Cedex 15, France
5. WHO Collaborating Centre for Research and Management on Zoonoses Control, Laboratoire d'Etudes sur la Rage & la Pathologie des Animaux Sauvages, Centre National d'Etudes Vétérinaires et alimentaires, Malzeville, France
6. WHO Collaborating Centre for Neurovirology, Department of Microbiology and Immunology, Thomas Jefferson University, Philadelphia, USA
7. WHO Collaborating Centre for Reference and Research on Rabies, Pasteur Institute of Iran, Teheran, Islamic Republic of Iran
8. WHO Collaborating Centre for Rabies Surveillance & Research, Institute of Epidemiology, Friedrich-Loeffler-Institut, Federal Research Institute for Animal Health, Wusterhausen, Germany

Box 7.2 (continued)

9. WHO Collaborating Centre for the Characterization of Rabies & Rabies-related Viruses, Veterinary Laboratories Agency – Weybridge, Department of Virology, Weybridge, Surrey, UK
10. WHO Collaborating Centre for Reference and Research in Rabies, Department of Neurovirology, National Institute of Mental Health and Neurosciences (NIMHANS), Bangalore, India
11. WHO Collaborating Centre for Rabies Epidemiology, National Institute of Communicable Diseases (National Centre for Disease Control), New Delhi, India
12. WHO Collaborating Centre for Research on Rabies Pathogenesis and Prevention, Queen Saovabha Memorial Institute, The Thai Red Cross Society, Bangkok, Thailand

Box 7.3 Reference Experts and Laboratories on Rabies (OIE 2013)

1. Dr. Christine Fehlner-Gardiner, Centre of Expertise for Rabies CFIA/ACIA, Ottawa Laboratory Fallowfield, Animal Diseases Research Institute, Nepean, Ontario, Canada
2. Prof. Changchun Tu, Diagnostic Laboratory for Rabies and Wildlife Associated Zoonoses, Department of Virology, Changchun Veterinary Research Institute (CVRI), Chinese Academy of Agricultural Sciences (CAAS), Changchun, Peoples Republic of China
3. Dr. Jacques Barrat and Dr. Florence Cliquet, Agence nationale de Sécurité Sanitaire de l'Alimentation, Laboratoire de la faune sauvage de Nancy, Malzéville Cedex, France
4. Dr. Thomas Müller, Institute for Epidemiology, Friedrich-Loeffler Institut,

(continued)

Box 7.3 (continued)

Federal Research Institute for Animal Health, Wusterhausen/Dosse, Germany

5. Dr. Dong-Kun Yang, Rabies Research Laboratory, Division of Viral Disease, Animal Plant and Fisheries Quarantine and Inspection Agency, Ministry of Food, Agriculture, Forestry and Fisheries, Gyeonggi, Republic of Korea
6. Dr. Claude Taurai Sabeta, Onderstepoort Veterinary Institute, Rabies Unit, Onderstepoort, South Africa
7. Dr. Anthony Fooks, Rabies and Wildlife Zoonoses Group, Virology Department, Animal Health and Veterinary Laboratories Agency, Surrey, Weybridge, UK
8. Dr Richard Franka, Poxvirus and Rabies Branch, Division of High-Consequence Pathogens and Pathology, National Center for Emerging and Zoonotic Infectious Diseases, Centers for Disease Control and Prevention, Atlanta, USA

7.7.3 Initiatives by the Global Alliance for Rabies Control

Global Alliance for Rabies Control (GARC, USA) and Alliance for Rabies Control (UK) are charitable, non-profit organisations. They took an initiative in 2006 to start World Rabies Day to undertake outreach programmes raising awareness about the impact of human and animal rabies and about the ease with which it can be prevented and eliminated. The inaugural campaign in September 2007 saw participation from nearly 400,000 people in 74 countries. Since then, it has seen much progress. World Rabies Day now involves every major human and animal health partner at the international, national, state/provincial, and local levels as well as veterinary, medical, and other specialised professional and student organisations, corporate, and non-profit partners, all working to mobilise awareness and resources in support of human rabies prevention and animal rabies control. Beginning in 2007 till the fifth anniversary of World Rabies Day in 2011, more than 2,000 events were held in 150 countries that helped in educating an estimated 182 million people and vaccinating 7.7 million animals (World Rabies Day 2012; GARC 2012a). World Rabies Day events are held in all sectors, from the ministries of health and agriculture to veterinary institutions and local groups. The campaigns facilitate political attention and support for rabies control.

GARC has also been instrumental in establishing and is a member of Partners for Rabies Prevention (GARC 2012a). This informal group includes all major international agencies involved in rabies, including the WHO, the Food and Agricultural Organization of the United Nations (FAO), the OIE, the WHO rabies collaborating centres, research scientists, representatives from the Bill and Melinda Gates Foundation, the UBS Optimus Foundation, and representatives from industry. A major achievement of this group is the preparation of Blueprint for Rabies Prevention, which has been written by world's foremost rabies experts (Partners for Rabies Prevention 2010). Available at www.rabiesblueprint.com free of cost to the governing bodies worldwide, it elaborates a roadmap and steps needed to reduce rabies.

In addition to this, GARC also works with the worldwide regional networks and management plans relating to rabies control (GARC 2012a). These include the Africa Rabies Expert Bureau (AfroREB), Asian Rabies Expert Bureau (AREB), North American Rabies Management Plan (NARMP), Middle East and Eastern Europe Rabies Expert Bureau (MEEREB), Meeting of Directors of National Programs for Rabies Control in all Latin American countries (REDIPRA), and Southern and Eastern African Rabies Group (SEARG).

7.8 Bottlenecks in Rabies Control

Many developed countries have successfully controlled dog rabies and even eliminated and human deaths due to rabies through extensive rabies control programmes; however, the situation in most of the developing countries remains grim. For example, despite having safe and effective modern rabies vaccines and great human resource, India continues to bear the greatest burden of rabies in the world. There are a number of factors that are responsible for slow progress or that may obstruct the implementation or success of action plans for rabies control and elimination. Several studies and analytical documents have dwelled upon these issues; the major constraints in rabies control are discussed below.

7.8.1 Lack of People's Perception of Rabies

A number of studies quite clearly show that people are generally deficient in understanding of various aspects of rabies, particularly in the developing countries. The attitude and practice still continue to be primitive, due to which the treatment options presently available are not property utilised. A survey by Agarwal and Reddaiah (2003) revealed that 40 % people exposed to animal bites did not seek any prophylaxis treatment.

Another study of 2,377 animal bite cases who attended the Anti-Rabies Clinic to seek postexposure advice and treatment in the city of Gwalior in India revealed that only 58.8 % persons reported to the clinic within 3 days of exposure, while the remaining were late with 13.9 % patients even reporting after 1 week. Of these, only 23.9 % of cases had taken some form of first aid measures like cleaning the wound with soap and water and applied some antiseptics while many others (46 %) had adopted some traditional kind of remedy like applying oil and pepper mixture on the wound (Agarwal and Mishra 2009).

A survey of 1,434 college students of Maddur town in Karnataka state in India revealed that only 46.4 % of them had the idea that rabies was caused by a virus. Although 97.6 % students were aware about transmission of rabies through dogs, only 53.1 % knew that the bite wound should immediately be washed with soap and water. The possibility of cats transmitting rabies was known to only 52.6 % students. Only 42.6 % students considered rabies as a 100 % fatal disease while only 44 % knew about the requirement of 5 doses of rabies vaccine by intramuscular route in case of an animal bite (Vinay and Mahendra 2009).

Ignorance about rabies prevention measures is rampant even among the people of excellent educational background. In an electronic survey of 100 persons from all over India, 90 % of the respondents agreed that dog bite wound should be washed with soap and water but the others did not have such perception. Seven per cent people even advocated the application of chilli powder on the bite wound (Garg 2009). Though 96 % persons knew about the requirement of antirabies vaccination after a street dog bite, there was widespread ignorance about the vaccination schedule. Only 68 % persons knew about it while 15 % people thought that a single injection would be sufficient. The remaining 17 % were not knowledgeable of the current vaccination regimens and still thought that 14 injections might still be necessary in bite cases. Only 32 % persons were aware that antirabies vaccination is given on the arm while the others indicated hip (32 %) or belly (36 %) as the sites of injection.

Pet dog owners also have poor knowledge about antirabies vaccination schedule in pet dogs. A recent survey carried out in Chandigarh in North India revealed that 18 % pet owners did not know the vaccination status of their dogs, while 66 % persons had got the initial immunisation done in their pets but subsequent annual boosters were not given (Singh et al. 2011).

Analysis of epidemiological and clinical features of 104 human rabies cases in Bali during 2008–2010 revealed that only 5.8 % had their wounds treated and received an antirabies vaccine after the bite incident. None of the patients received RIG (Susilawathi et al. 2012). The study indicated that human fatalities occurred because of lack of knowledge regarding rabies risk, poor management of dog bites, and limited availability of RIG. The situation in Cambodia is also similar. A study in an urban and peri-urban province of the country showed that though 93.2 % (233/250) of the respondents had heard of the disease rabies, but only 77.3 % (180/233) of these persons knew it was fatal to humans. Further, only 51.9 % (121/233) of them were aware of the vaccine for dogs (Lunney et al. 2012).

7.8.2 Physicians' Inadequate Knowledge

Studies reveal that a large number of medical personnel have inadequate knowledge about wound management practices and administration of antirabies vaccine and RIG. In many cases, the antirabies vaccine is administered in a wrong site (gluteal muscle) while RIG is not administered at all despite that it is indicated according to the guidelines. In a study of animal bite cases coming to Anti-Rabies Clinic in Gwalior in India, it was revealed that a vast majority of the patients (57.7 %), who had previously taken treatment at other places, were given antirabies vaccine shots over the gluteal region while RIG had not been administered in any of these cases (Agarwal and Mishra 2009). In another study of clinical profile of 945 children attending Anti-Rabies Clinic at Berhampur in India for PEP, Pratap et al. (2009) observed that 875 (92 %) children had Category III exposure but their local medical attendants had not administered RIG to any of them. Moreover, majority of the children had been given antirabies vaccine injections over the gluteal region.

A recent study revealed many gaps in the knowledge and practices concerning animal bite management among the doctors working in government hospitals, dispensaries, and private settings in New Delhi. Of them, 81.4 % were conversant with the PEP schedule in unimmunised patients, but only 40.4 % knew about the postexposure schedule in previously immunised patients, and only 47.8 % had the idea of the pre-exposure prophylaxis schedule (Garg et al. 2012). Only a small proportion of the doctors knew the correct intradermal rabies prophylaxis schedule (39.1 %), site (42.2 %), and dose (48.4 %). Another recent study focussing on the evaluation of knowledge of zoonoses among medical students and recent graduates revealed critical gaps in medical education with respect to zoonoses. Out of 364 respondents, only 10 defined zoonoses accurately (2.8 %). Only 5.5 % of the persons were able to identify rabies as a disease transmitted by animals other than dogs (Kakkar et al. 2011).

Similar deficiencies in the correct perception regarding animal wound management and vaccine administration have been observed among the general practitioners in India's neighbouring country Pakistan. In an evaluation of 151 general practitioners in Karachi, 77.5 % of them knew the cause of rabies, but only 51.7 % were knowledgeable about the incubation period of rabies (Shah et al. 2009). Only 19.4 % of the clinicians had appropriate idea of the first-line treatment, while almost all of them (98 %) had no knowledge about the types of antirabies vaccine. Only 19.2 % of them knew about antirabies serum.

A survey of 890 Turkish physicians revealed their insufficient basic and clinical knowledge of rabies (Gonen et al. 2011). The average score of the physicians was 64.5 ± 16 and that for clinical rabies knowledge was 62.8 ± 12 out of 100; however, 68 % of them were not aware of the proper method for cleaning wounds as a first-line treatment in PEP. In addition, 38.4 % physicians did not understand the administration of vaccines together with immunoglobulin as part of PEP. The study also showed that 79 % physicians did not know the correct doses of vaccines, while 37.6 % did not know the correct sites and routes of vaccine administration. Finally, 30 % physicians were not aware of the correct PEP vaccine schedules.

7.8.3 Short Supply of Vaccines and Other Resources

Safe and efficacious rabies biologicals are in critical short supply globally, particularly RIG. According to a survey, the annual incidence of animal bites in India is estimated at 17.4 million (APCRI 2004); however, the vaccine utilisation data indicate that only about five million people receive PEP (Mittal 2009). Apparently, a large number of people suffering animal bites do not get postexposure treatment which is the key to prevention of rabies. Apart from ignorance, poverty and inadequate financial resources of health departments may be a major hurdle in the people's access to rabies prophylaxis. The unavailability of adequate medical facilities, particularly in rural and remote areas, also worsens the situation. The availability of RIG is a real challenge as it may not be readily available even in big towns in developing countries.

7.8.4 Poor Resources for Dog Rabies Control

Control of rabies in dogs constitutes an integral part of rabies control programme. Extensive efforts have largely controlled dog rabies in many developed countries but it remains enzootic in much of the developing world including India. In a recent study on 100 street dogs and 50 household dogs in Chandigarh, a state capital and modern city in India, the protective titre of antirabies antibodies in serum (0.5 IU/ml) was detected only in 1 % of street dogs and 16 % of pet dogs (Singh et al. 2011). The unavailability of sufficient resources (vaccine, funds, manpower) and lack of organised programmes and strict legislations are the reasons for the grim situation.

7.8.5 Neglect of Stray Animal Management

Stray dogs act as the principal reservoir of rabies in developing countries. According to estimates, the pet, owned, and household dog population in India is around 28 million (APCRI 2004). Dog bites are the most common cause of human rabies infection in Asia and Africa, which carry the greatest burden of human and animal deaths due to rabies. The increase in human cases is linked to the proliferation of roaming dogs, which include not only stray dogs but also the owned dogs. Lack of systematic approach for successful dog population management is usually responsible for uncontrolled increase in the dog population resulting in more chances of exposing human beings and livestock to rabies.

At some places, where dog reproduction control programmes are in operation, these may not be dealing with the issue to a desired level due to prohibitive cost considerations. The average cost for the medicines and consumables per surgical sterilisation in developing countries has been found to be US$7.50 which may vary from US$3 to US$315 depending upon the country. The full costs (including veterinarians and veterinary support staff, clinic running costs, all medicines, and consumables) may range from US$10 to US$352, with an average of US$30 per sterilisation (Partners for Rabies Prevention 2010). Development of cheaper safe and effective contraceptives and sterilants may help in greater success of animal birth control campaigns.

7.8.6 Missing Political Commitment

Effective implementation of rabies control programmes may not be possible without a strong political will despite the availability of biologicals, scientific methods, community participation, and financial resources. As the success of rabies control programmes is influenced by multiple sectors, it requires widespread commitment at national and regional levels among the ministries and departments concerning public health, animal health, wildlife, forests, environment, finance, law and justice, local civic bodies, and education.

7.8.7 Inadequate Disease Surveillance and Laboratory Facilities

Poorly developed disease surveillance system and scarce diagnostic facilities in developing countries pose great difficulty in proper risk analysis and evaluation of disease control programmes. Similarly, inadequate laboratory facilities for evaluation of efficacy and quality assurance of vaccines and immunoglobulin threaten the developing countries with the problem of PEP failure.

7.8.8 Weak Intersectoral Coordination

Human beings and animals, including domestic animal species and wildlife species, are inextricably linked in the transmission cycle of rabies. However, collaboration between different sectors including public health and animal health is usually very weak or even absent in many cases. This probably is the major reason for slow progress in rabies control. Involvement and coordinated functioning of public health agencies, veterinary organisations, wildlife department, and civic bodies is essential for the success of rabies control programmes.

7.8.9 Lack of Public Cooperation

The cooperation of people is inevitable for the success of any public health programme including rabies control programmes. However, due to widespread illiteracy, ignorance, and financial constraints, the participation of people in the developing countries is usually not up to the desired level. For example, in India, irresponsible pet ownership is rampant resulting in unrestricted movements and unvaccinated status of even the pet dogs. People due to their cultural and religious beliefs engage in feeding stray animals. Moreover, the practice of disposing household and kitchen waste in open is not uncommon which attracts the stray dogs and brings them near to the human habitations. Inadequate public support leads to poor results of any public health programme.

7.8.10 Myths and Religious Factors Among the Community

Due to the widespread prevalence of myths, blind faiths, and certain religious factors, particularly in rural and remote areas, many victims of animal bites do not seek medical advice promptly. In animal bite cases, the recourse to indigenous treatment (45.3 %) and application of local remedies to wound (36.8 %) is quite prevalent (Sudarshan et al. 2006). In a study of 24 clinically diagnosed and reported rabies cases encountered in the Anti-Rabies Clinic of a medical college in Orissa (Odisha) during a 4-year study period, 79 % had not taken any antirabies treatment, while all of them had undergone treatment by traditional systems of medicine (Satapathy et al. 2005).

It is a common practice in the rural household to apply chilli powder on the bite wounds (Agarwal and Mishra 2009). A survey by Agarwal and Reddaiah (2003) revealed that half of the people exposed to animal bites applied chilli powder to the affected parts immediately after the bite. Some bite victims also apply salt, turmeric powder, lime, snuff powder, paste of leaves, acid, etc. Some people seek remedies from religious places and local saints and apply holy ash to the bite wounds (Ichhpujani et al. 2008). These practices may vary from one region to another. As a result, these people lose precious time and put their lives to risk by depending on home remedies alone.

7.9 The Way Forward

In spite of wide prevalence and fatal nature of rabies and the availability of scientific preventive and control methods, the disease remains largely neglected or attracts low priority, particularly in the developing world. Financial resource crunch and lack of commitment at the local, national, regional, and global levels are the major reasons for the grim situation; however, these constraints need to be overcome through cost-effective technological advancements. Improved surveillance systems are also essential to get realistic data for better advocacy of rabies control programmes.

A number of approaches for effective control of rabies have been elaborately defined. It is imperative to integrate and apply the best suited options and combination according to the situational backgrounds as their applicability and efficacy may vary in different settings. Strategic implementation, multisectoral coordination, people's participation, and continuous evaluation are the keys to success of the rabies control programmes and should not be missed.

References

Afya (2012) About the Afya Serengeti project. http://www.afya.org/project.asp. Accessed 5 July 2012

Agarwal AK, Mishra A (2009) Demographic characteristics of animal bite cases attending the anti rabies clinic of G. R. Medical College Hospital, Gwalior (Madhya Pradesh). Souvenir, 11th national conference of the association for prevention and control of rabies in

India, Thiruvananthapuram, July 4–5, 2009, p 28. http://rabies.org.in/rabies/wp-content/uploads/2009/11/APCRICON-2009-Souvenir.pdf. Accessed 5 July 2012

Agarwal N, Reddaiah VP (2003) Knowledge, attitude and practice following dog bite: a community-based epidemiological study. Health Popul Perspect Issues 26(4):154–161

APCRI (2004) Assessing burden of rabies in India, WHO sponsored national multi-centric rabies survey 2003, Final report. Association for Prevention and Control of Rabies in India. www.apcri.org. Accessed 11 June 2012

APCRI (2006) Rabies prophylaxis guidelines. Association for Prevention and Control of Rabies in India. http://rabies.org.in/rabies/wp-content/uploads/2009/11/APCRI-Guidelines-for-Rabies-Prophylaxis.pdf. Accessed 11 June 2012

AWBI (2009) Standard operating procedures for sterilization of stray dogs under the animal birth control programme. Animal Welfare Board of India, Chennai

Belotto A, Leanes LF, Schneider MC, Tamayo H, Correa E (2005) Overview of rabies in Americas. Virus Res 111:5–12

CDC (2012) Rabies. Centers for Disease Control and Prevention. http://www.cdc.gov/rabies/. Accessed 30 Mar 2012

Cliquet F, Gurbuxani JP, Pradhan HK, Pattnaik B, Patil SS, Regnault A, Begouen H, Guiot AL, Sood R, Mahl P, Singh R, Meslin FX, Picard E, Aubert MF, Barrat J (2007) The safety and efficacy of the oral rabies vaccine SAG2 in Indian stray dogs. Vaccine 25:3409–3418

Dodet B, Goswami A, Gunasekera A, de Guzman F, Jamali S, Montalban C, Purba W, Quiambao B, Salahuddin N, Sampath G, Tang Q, Tantawichien T, Wimalaratne O, Ziauddin A (2008) Rabies awareness in eight Asian countries. Vaccine 26:6344–6348

Estrada R, Vos A, Leon RD, Mueller T (2001) Field trial with oral vaccination of dogs against rabies in the Philippines. BMC Infect Dis 1:23

GARC (2012a) Global alliance for rabies control. http://www.rabiescontrol.net/. Accessed 5 July 2012

GARC (2012b) The Bohol rabies prevention and elimination project wins the Galing Pook. Global alliance for rabies control. http://www.rabiescontrol.net/what-we-do/project-reports.html. Accessed 5 July 2012

Garg SR (2009). Rabies awareness among literate people in India. Souvenir, national symposium and VIII annual conference of Indian Association of Veterinary Public Health Specialists, Gangtok, 6–7 Nov 2009, p 34

Garg SR (2012) Strategies for elimination of rabies. In: Garg SR (ed) Veterinary and livestock sector: a blueprint for capacity building. Satish Serial Publishing House, Delhi, pp 273–307

Garg A, Kumar R, Ingle GK (2012) Knowledge and practices regarding animal bite management and rabies prophylaxis among doctors in Delhi, India. Asia Pac J Public Health. doi:10.1177/1010539511436323

GOI (2001) Animal Birth Control (Dogs) Rules, 2001. Gazette of India, extraordinary notification number S.O. 1256(E) dated 24th Dec, 2001. Government of India, New Delhi. http://www.moef.nic.in/legis/awbi/awbi13.html

GOI (2011) Animal Birth Control (Dogs) Amendment Rules, 2010. Gazette of India, Notification number S.O. 303(E) dated 8th Feb 2011. Ministry of Environment and Forests, Government of India, New Delhi. http://www.moef.nic.in//downloads/rules-and-regulations/303-E.pdf

Gonen I, Soysal A, Topuzoglu A, Bakir M (2011) Clinical knowledge and attitudes of Turkish physicians toward rabies caused by animal bites. Jpn J Infect Dis 64:382–390

Hanlon CA, Childs JE, Nettles VF, National Working Group on Rabies Prevention and Control (1999) Recommendations of the working group on rabies. Article III: rabies in wildlife. J Am Vet Med Assoc 215:1612–1618

Ichhpujani RL, Mala C, Veena M, Singh J, Bhardwaj M, Bhattacharya D, Pattanaik SK, Balakrishnan N, Reddy AK, Samnpath G, Gandhi N, Nagar SS, Shiv L (2008) Epidemiology of animal bites and rabies cases in India. A multicentric study. J Commun Dis 40(1):27–36

Kakkar M, Ramani S, Menon G, Sankhe L, Gaidhane A, Krishnan S (2011) Zoonoses? Not sure what that is. An assessment of knowledge of zoonoses among medical students in India. Trans R Soc Trop Med Hyg 105:254–261

Knobel DL, Cleaveland S, Coleman PG, Fevre EM, Meltzer MI, Miranda ME, Shaw A, Zinsstag J, Meslin FX (2005) Re-evaluating the burden of rabies in Africa and Asia. Bull WHO 83:360–368

Lucas CH, Pino FV, Baer G, Morales PK, Cedillo VG, Blanco MA, Avila MH (2008) Rabies control in Mexico. Dev Biol (Basel) 131:167–175

Lunney M, Fèvre SJS, Stiles E, Ly S, San S, Vong S (2012) Knowledge, attitudes and practices of rabies prevention and dog bite injuries in urban and peri-urban provinces in Cambodia, 2009. Int Health 4:4–9

Mittal V (2009) Burning issues in rabies control in India. Souvenir, 11th national conference of the Association for Prevention and Control of Rabies in India (APCRI), Thiruvananthapuram, 4–5 July 2009, pp 7–9. http://rabies.org.in/rabies/wp-content/uploads/2009/11/APCRICON-2009-Souvenir.pdf. Accessed 5 July 2012

Müller T, Freuling CM (2011) Rabies elimination in Europe – a success story. OIE Global conference on rabies control: Towards sustainable prevention at the source, 7–9 Sept 2011, Incheon-Seoul, Korea. http://www.oie.int/eng/A_RABIES/Abstracts_rabiesConf/abstract1-6/S1-2/M%C3%BCller%20T.pdf. Accessed 6 July 2012

OIE (2009) Eliminating rabies in dogs is the optimal control method for preventing spread of the disease. Press release, World Organisation for Animal Health, Paris, 13 Mar 2009. http://www.oie.int. Accessed 12 May 2011

OIE (2011) Terrestrial animal health code, Chapter 7.7 Stray dog population control. World Organisation for Animal Health, Paris. http://www.oie.int/fileadmin/Home/eng/Health_standards/tahc/2010/en_chapitre_1.7.7.htm. Accessed 28 June 2012

OIE (2013) Reference experts and laboratories. World Organisation for Animal Health. http://www.oie.int/en/our-scientific-expertise/reference-laboratories/list-of-laboratories/. Accessed 5 June 2013

PAHO (2012) Elimination of dog-transmitted human rabies in Latin America: Situation analysis. Pan American Health Organization, Washington, DC. http://www.paho.org/English/AD/DPC/VP/rabia-sit.htm#fin. Accessed 5 July 2012

Partners for Rabies Prevention (2010) Blueprint for rabies prevention and control. http://www.rabiesblueprint.com/. Accessed 12 Apr 2012

Perera MA, Harischandra PA, Wimalaratne O, Damboragama SN (2000) Feasibility of canine oral rabies vaccination in Sri Lanka – a preliminary report. Ceylon Med J 45(2):61–64

Pratap AK, Behera TR, Malini DS, Satapathy DM, Tripathy RM (2009) Clinical profile of children attending ARC, MKCG Medical College, Behrampur. Souvenir, 11th national conference of the Association for Prevention and Control of Rabies in India (APCRI), Thiruvananthapuram, 4–5 July 2009, p 30. http://rabies.org.in/rabies/wp-content/uploads/2009/11/APCRICON-2009-Souvenir.pdf. Accessed 5 July 2012

Rabies Bulletin Europe (2012) Rabies information system of the WHO collaboration centre for Rabies Surveillance and Research. http://www.who-rabies-bulletin.org. Accessed 8 Apr 2012

Rabiesblueprint (2012) Successful rabies control in KwaZulu Natal. http://www.rabiesblueprint.com/Successful-rabies-control-in. Accessed 5 July 2012

Rosatte R (2011) Evolution of wildlife rabies control tactics. Adv Virus Res 79:397–419

Rupprecht CE, Stohr K, Meredith C (2001) Rabies. In: Williams ES, Barker IK (eds) Infectious diseases of wild mammals. Iowa State University Press, Ames, pp 3–36

Satapathy DM, Sahu T, Behera TR, Patnaik JK, Malini DS (2005) Socio-clinical profile of rabies cases in anti-rabies clinic, M. K. C. G. Medical College, Orissa. Indian J Public Health 49:241–242

Schneider MC, Belotto A, Adé MP, Leanes LF, Correa E, Tamayo H, Medina G, Rodrigues MJ (2005) Epidemiologic situation of human rabies in Latin America in 2004. Epidemiol Bull/PAHO 26(1):2–4

Shah SF, Jawed M, Nooruddin S, Afzal S, Sajid F, Majeed S, Naveed M, Mustafa K, Azhar M (2009) Knowledge and practices among the general practitioners of Karachi regarding dog bite management. J Pak Med Assoc 59:861–864

Singh MP, Goyal K, Majumdar M, Ratho RK (2011) Prevalence of rabies antibodies in street and household dogs in Chandigarh, India. Trop Anim Health Prod 43:111–114

Smith TG, Wu X, Franka R, Rupprecht CE (2011) Design of future rabies biologics and antiviral drugs. Adv Virus Res 79:345–363

Sudarshan MK, Mahendra BJ, Madhusudana SN, Ashwath Narayana DH, Rahman A, Rao NS, X-Meslin F, Lobo D, Ravikumar K, Gangaboraiah (2006) An epidemiological study of animal bites in India: results of a WHO sponsored national multi-centric rabies survey. J Commun Dis 38(1):32–39

Susilawathi NM, Darwinata AE, Dwija IB, Budayanti NS, Wirasandhi GAK, Subrata K, Susilarini NK, Sudewi RAA, Wignall FS, Mahardika GNK (2012) Epidemiological and clinical features of human rabies cases in Bali 2008–2010. BMC Infect Dis 12:81

Tamayo H, Cosivi O, Vigilato M, Valderrama W (2011) Elimination of human rabies transmitted by dogs in the Latin America and the Caribbeans: Achievements. OIE Global conference on rabies control: Towards sustainable prevention at the source, 7–9 Sept 2011, Incheon-Seoul, Korea. http://www.oie.int/eng/A_RABIES/Abstracts_rabiesConf/abstract1-6/S1-2/Tamayo%20H.pdf. Accessed 5 July 2012

Taylor L, Romijn P (2012) São Paulo has a case of animal rabies after 30 years. Rabid Bytes Issue 26, Feb 2012, Global alliance for rabies control. www.rabiescontrol.net. Accessed 18 Aug 2012

USDA (2012) National Rabies Management Program. Animal and Plant Health Inspection Service, United States Department of Agriculture. http://www.aphis.usda.gov/ws/rabies/vaccine.html. Accessed 1 July 2012

Vinay M, Mahendra BJ (2009) Effectiveness of 'awareness sessions' for enhancing knowledge regarding rabies among college students. Souvenir, 11th National Conference of the Association for Prevention and Control of Rabies in India (APCRI), Thiruvananthapuram, 2009, p 35. http://rabies.org.in/rabies/wp-content/uploads/2009/11/APCRICON-2009-Souvenir.pdf. Accessed 5 July 2012

WHO (2001) Strategies for the control and elimination of rabies in Asia. Report of a WHO Interregional Consultation Geneva, 17–21 July 2001. World Health Organization, Department of Communicable Disease Surveillance and Response, WHO/CDS/CSR/EPH/2002.8

WHO (2005) WHO Expert Consultation on Rabies. First report. WHO Technical Report Series, No. 931. World Health Organization, Geneva

WHO (2007) Oral vaccination of dogs against rabies. Guidance for research on oral rabies vaccines and field application of oral vaccination of dogs against rabies. World Health Organization, Geneva

WHO (2008) Rabies in the South-East Asia region. World Health Organization, New Delhi

WHO (2010) Rabies vaccines: WHO position paper. Wkly Epidemiol Rec 32(85):309–320

WHO (2012a) Current strategies for human rabies pre and post-exposure prophylaxis. Guide for post-exposure prophylaxis (PEP). http://www.who.int/rabies/human/WHO_strategy_prepost_exposure/en/index1.html. Accessed 15 Aug 2012

WHO (2012b) Rabies. World Health Organization. www.who.int. Accessed 10 Mar 2012

WHO SEARO (2012) Rabies: Country profile: India. World Health Organization, Regional Office for South-East Asia, New Delhi. http://www.searo.who.int/LinkFiles/Zoonoses_IND-rabies-cp.pdf. Accessed 15 Aug 2012

Wilde H (2007) Failures of rabies post-exposure prophylaxis. Vaccine 25:7605–7609

World Rabies Day (2012) http://www.worldrabiesday.org/. Accessed 5 July 2012

Zhang S, Liu Y, Fooks AR, Zhang F, Hu R (2008) Oral vaccination of dogs (*Canis familiaris*) with baits containing the recombinant rabies-canine adenovirus type-2 vaccine confers long-lasting immunity against rabies. Vaccine 26(3):345–350

8 Frequently Asked Questions

Abstract

Rabies is a serious viral disease that occurs in all mammals including humans. Domestic and pet animals affected with the disease include dogs, cats, ferrets, horses, cows, buffaloes, sheep, goats, camels etc. Wild animals that are most at risk include mongooses, foxes, wolves, raccoons, skunks, groundhogs, coyotes, bobcats, beavers, fishers, minks, otters, muskrats, and bats in some regions. Rabies has very wide prevalence across the world and kills more than 50,000 people and millions of animals every year. The disease is endemic in India. Despite being vaccine preventable, rabies continues to kill primarily due to rampant ignorance and people's wrong perceptions of the disease. Many times even healthcare personnel and veterinarians have doubts about the actions required in individual cases of suspected exposures for prevention of rabies as well as for their own safeguard against the occupational risk. This chapter presents 200 frequently asked questions and attempts to clear the doubts of the people of all strata of the community including pet lovers, public health professionals, veterinarians, and the common people concerning the risk of rabies and preventive measures in different situations.

1. **What is rabies?**
   Rabies is a serious disease that can infect mammals. It causes inflammation of the brain. Once symptoms begin, there is no treatment for rabies, and it is always fatal. In man, the disease is also known as hydrophobia (fear of water).
2. **What causes rabies?**
   Rabies is caused by a virus that affects mammals, including humans. Sick animals can transmit the disease through their saliva, either by biting or through direct contact between saliva and broken skin or mucous membranes. Rabies virus can then travel through nerves to the brain where it causes inflammation and the symptoms of rabies appear.
3. **Which animals can get rabies?**
   All mammals, including humans, can become infected with the rabies viruses. Domestic animals and pets such as dogs, cats, ferrets, horses, cows, buffaloes, sheep,

S.R. Garg, *Rabies in Man and Animals*, DOI 10.1007/978-81-322-1605-6_8,

goats, and camels can also be infected. Wild animals that are most at risk include mongooses, foxes, wolves, raccoons, skunks, groundhogs, coyotes, bobcats, beavers, fishers, minks, otters, muskrats, and bats in some regions. Rodents and rabbits are much less likely to carry rabies. Birds, reptiles, amphibians, and fish do not become infected.

4. **How serious is rabies?**
   Rabies is an extremely painful and deadly disease. If prompt and appropriate postexposure treatment is not received, the disease is fatal. Rabies kills about 50,000 people around the world each year.
5. **Is rabies prevalent throughout the world?**
   Rabies has very wide prevalence across the world. Only in few countries it has not been reported.
6. **How common is rabies in the world?**
   Rabies is a big problem in Asia, Africa, and Central and South America. Each year, rabies kills more than 50,000 people and millions of animals worldwide. Exposure to rabid dogs is the cause of over 90 % of human rabies cases. Rabies is encountered everywhere except in few countries. In some regions, rabies has been almost eliminated from domestic dogs, but the virus is still active in the wildlife population.
7. **What is the status of rabies in India?**
   Rabies is endemic in India. The cases of rabies in animals occur frequently in the country; hence, chances of human exposure are very high. The largest number of human deaths due to rabies occurs in India.
8. **What is the extent of human rabies in India?**
   It is estimated that more than 20,000 human deaths occur due to rabies in India annually.
9. **Is rabies prevalent everywhere in India?**
   Rabies is widely prevalent in India but Andaman, Nicobar, and Lakshadweep islands are free of rabies.
10. **Which animals are reservoirs of rabies infection in India?**
    Dogs, cats, mongoose, foxes, jackals, and other wild animals are major reservoirs. The rabies virus maintains itself in such reservoir animals.
11. **How is rabies prevented?**
    There are vaccines that are effective in preventing rabies. In humans, rabies can be prevented by reducing exposure to unvaccinated animals, unfamiliar animals, and wild or exotic animals. In case of exposure to a potentially rabid animal, there is a postexposure prophylaxis (PEP) treatment which, when administered appropriately, can prevent the disease in exposed persons.
12. **What should I do if I am bitten by an animal?**
    Thoroughly cleanse the bite wound with soap and water. Next, you should immediately seek medical attention. Appropriate wound care and the need for PEP treatment will be determined by your healthcare provider. If possible, the animal should be safely confined for observation or examination for rabies.
13. **What is the incidence of dog bites in India?**
    It is estimated that annually there are 17 million cases of animal bites in India, more than 90 % of which are due to dogs.
14. **What are the most dangerous sites of bite exposure in man?**
    The bites on the body parts with more nerve supply like head, neck, face, hands, and genitals are more dangerous, though infection may occur at any bite wound site.
15. **Is there any treatment for rabies?**
    There is no treatment for rabies once a person or animal manifests the signs of disease. Death is inevitable in such cases. However, rabies can be prevented by taking timely and appropriate PEP after an exposure to rabies.
16. **What happens if a person develops rabies?**
    Rabies is fatal. Clinical rabies management is almost universally futile and treatment is only supportive.
17. **How is rabies transmitted to humans?**
    People usually get rabies from the bite of a rabid animal. However, it is also possible to get the infection if infectious material

from a rabid animal, such as saliva, enters directly into eyes, nose, mouth, or a wound.

18. **What are the factors that influence transmission of rabies virus and occurrence of disease in man after a rabid dog bite?**
Amount of saliva, concentration of virus, strain of virus at the bite wound site, the site of bite (nearness to head), severity of bite, and the number, size, and depth of bite wounds are some important factors that influence the transmission of rabies virus.

19. **What are the factors that influence protection against rabies after a dog bite?**
The type of wound care immediately after the bite (washing of wound, application of antiseptics), prompt and adequate vaccination, site of vaccine injection, potency of vaccine, and application of rabies immunoglobulin (RIG) are the major factors that decide the protection against rabies.

20. **Can I get rabies in any other way than an animal bite?**
Non-bite exposures to rabies may occur due to scratches and exposure of abrasions, open wounds, or mucous membranes to saliva or other potentially infectious material (such as brain tissue) from a rabid animal. Inhalation of aerosolised rabies virus is also a potential route of exposure, particularly among the laboratory workers.

21. **Does a vaccinated dog pose risk of rabies?**
Modern tissue culture veterinary vaccines are efficacious. The pets getting the vaccination regularly are generally considered protected. However, ideally, the protective antibody level in the pet's blood should be tested to ensure efficacy of the vaccine but this is generally not done. Consequently, to avoid the risk, a bite even by a vaccinated dog in rabies-endemic areas like India should be considered as a suspected case and should not be ignored. The postexposure immunisation should be initiated in the bitten person immediately. Simultaneously, the dog is kept under observation for 10 days. If the dog remains healthy for 10 days after the bite, further vaccination may then be discontinued.

22. **Can a pet dog also be rabid?**
Yes.

23. **What is a street virus?**
Street virus is virulent. It has long and variable incubation period of about 3 weeks to 3 months.

24. **What is fixed virus?**
Fixed virus is an attenuated street virus. It is least virulent and has a fixed short incubation period of 5–9 days. It is used for making vaccines.

25. **What is the risk of rabies from squirrels, mice, rats and, other rodents?**
Small rodents (such as squirrels, rats, mice, hamsters, guinea pigs, gerbils, and chipmunks) and lagomorphs (such as rabbits and hares) are almost never found to be infected with rabies and have not been known to cause rabies among humans. Bites by these animals are usually not considered a risk of rabies unless the animal was sick or behaving in any unusual manner and rabies is widespread in the area. However, woodchucks or groundhogs have been reported to carry the infection in USA.

26. **Does the age of biting dog influence rabies transmission?**
No. Age, size, breed, or sex of the dog does not influence transmission of rabies.

27. **If a rabid dog bites a healthy dog, and the next day this dog bites a person, what should be done?**
The dog may not develop rabies within a day; however, the earlier status of the apparently healthy dog is not known. Vaccination may therefore be done for safety.

28. **Does an unvaccinated pet dog pose danger to the pet owner?**
In the rabies enzootic areas, unvaccinated pet dog may develop rabies if bitten by a stray dog, thus, posing threat to the pet owner and his family members and visitors.

29. **Can rabies be transmitted by feeding street dogs?**
No. Rabies cannot be transmitted just by the nearness of the dogs unless the dog bites a person or licks his broken skin.

30. **On a camping trip in USA, we woke up to find a bat in our tent. Does it constitute a rabies risk?**
Yes, because bat rabies is prevalent in USA. Bats have small teeth and claws, so bite marks may be very small that may go unnoticed. Therefore, you should consult a doctor as soon as possible regarding postexposure rabies vaccination.
31. **Is bat rabies present in India?**
No. It is not reported.
32. **Can milk from a rabid animal contain rabies virus?**
In theory, it is possible for rabies virus to be transmitted via milk, but there are very few published reports about the presence of rabies virus in cow milk.
33. **Is there any risk of rabies due to consumption of milk of a rabid cow, buffalo, goat, etc.? Does such person require vaccination?**
Boiling or adequate heating of milk kills the rabies virus. However, if raw milk or milk product has been consumed or when a person is not sure about whether the milk was adequately heated or not, he may be advised to undergo vaccination.
34. **Can people become infected with rabies by drinking unpasteurised milk?**
In theory, it is possible for someone to become infected with rabies by drinking raw milk from an infected animal. However, there are no documented reports of such cases.
35. **Can rabies be transmitted through food (by eating milk or meat)?**
Rabies virus is killed by heating; therefore pasteurised milk or cooked meat does not cause an exposure. However, drinking unpasteurised milk from a rabid cow or goat is considered an exposure.
36. **Can rabies be transmitted while slaughtering animals?**
Exposure to rabies as a result of butchering, processing, or consuming a rabid animal is possible. Butchering of unvaccinated dogs and cats, for example, has been recognised as an increasing human health risk in countries where consumption of dog and cat meat is undertaken (e.g. in some Asian countries). Exposure to rabies virus can occur through contamination of cuts or abrasions or consumption of infected brain. Exposure can be prevented by wearing protective clothing and avoiding consumption of uncooked meat.
37. **Can I get rabies due to sharing food and water with a patient who had rabies?**
It is unlikely that rabies will be transmitted through sharing food and water, but if saliva from the infected patient comes in contact with your mucous membranes (mouth), then this would be an exposure and you should seek treatment.
38. **Is raccoon rabies or bat rabies more dangerous than the rabies caused by dogs?**
The disease itself is the same, only the reservoir hosts may be different in different geographical areas.
39. **Does rabies infection occur through air?**
In some countries, bats are known to transmit rabies infection. The rabies virus may be present in the air in caves where bats are present. Cases of human rabies have been reported through aerosol (inhalation of contaminated air) in persons going to such caves. It can also occur accidentally in rabies vaccine and research laboratories.
40. **Does a person suffering from rabies excrete rabies virus in saliva?**
Yes, the saliva of a person suffering from rabies carries virus and can transmit infection.
41. **Can rabies be transmitted from one person to another?**
Few cases of rabies caused by human-to-human transmission have been reported through cornea and organ transplants. Bite and non-bite exposures inflicted by infected humans could theoretically transmit rabies, but no such cases have been documented. Casual contact, such as touching a person with rabies or contact with non-infectious fluid or tissue (urine, blood, faeces), does not constitute an exposure and does not require PEP.
42. **Can a hydrophobic patient transmit infection through kissing?**
Rabies virus is present in the saliva of a hydrophobic patient. Kissing, therefore,

can transmit the infection to the other person through injuries or ulcers in the mouth.

43. **Can rabies be transmitted through sexual intercourse?**
Rabies virus is present in the semen and to some extent in vaginal secretions of hydrophobic patients. Hence, sexual intercourse can transmit infection.

44. **I have had contact with a person who is undergoing rabies vaccination after a dog bite. Could this person transmit rabies to me? Should I receive postexposure vaccination?**
A healthy person undergoing postexposure vaccination after a potential exposure does not pose a rabies risk to others. A person receives rabies vaccination to prevent the occurrence of rabies after exposure. You do not need vaccination because that person does not have rabies.

45. **I have heard that rabies patients are infectious before they show signs of illness. What is the length of time that they are infectious before becoming ill?**
The infectious period in human beings before the appearance of clinical sign is not fully clear. Domestic animals, such as cats and dogs, have rabies virus present in their saliva only a few days before the onset of clinical signs. Other animals may have virus in their saliva longer. Because the infectious period is not fully known for humans, public health officials are recommending that anyone who had non-intact skin or mucous membrane contact with saliva or who has received transplant from the donor within 14 days before and anytime after the patient's onset of illness should receive PEP.

46. **I visited a hospital where a rabies patient was treated. Am I at risk for rabies?**
No, in such circumstances you would not have been exposed to rabies, there is no risk of rabies exposure to you.

47. **I am a healthcare worker. I handled rabies-infected organs for a transplant procedure in the hospital. Am I at risk for rabies?**
Healthcare workers who may have handled an organ to be transplanted are at low risk for exposure because the virus is contained within the nerve tissue of the organ. However, certain procedures that might generate sprays or splashes containing nerve tissue theoretically pose a risk for exposure to the rabies virus. Safety measures such as using gowns, gloves, mask, goggles, or face shield would prevent such exposure. In case of an exposure, rabies PEP would be recommended.

48. **I am a healthcare worker. I took care of a rabies patient after or shortly before he developed clinical signs of rabies. Am I at risk for rabies?**
There are no known cases of rabies transmission to healthcare workers caring for patients with rabies. Any bite from a human rabies patient is an obvious exposure to rabies. Non-bite exposure may occur due to contamination of open wounds, abrasions, or mucous membranes with saliva or other potentially infectious material (such as neural tissue and other innervated tissue) from a rabid human. Other contact, such as touching a rabid human and contact with blood, urine, cerebrospinal fluid, or faeces of a rabid human, does not constitute an exposure. However, an accident with sharp instruments or needles (a penetrating wound from a contaminated sharp instrument) or lack of personal protective equipment may cause contamination of mucous membrane or non-intact skin with potentially infectious material (droplet splashes to the eyes, nose, or mouth). Adherence to standard precautions will minimise the risk of exposure.

49. **Under what circumstances a healthcare worker taking care of a human rabies patient should seek PEP?**
Healthcare workers who had an open wound, non-intact skin, or mucous membrane contact with a patient's saliva or other potentially infectious material and those who experienced an injury with a contaminated needle, scalpel, or other sharp device related to patient care should receive rabies PEP.

50. **Why is a needle stick injury considered a rabies exposure if the virus is not present in the blood?**
Infectious nerve material could be contained in the bore of the needle following tissue penetration in a rabies patient. Thus, there may be the possibility of exposure due to nerve tissue rather than blood exposure.

51. **What are the circumstances in healthcare settings that are not a risk for rabies exposure?**
Exposure to faeces, urine, blood, or other body fluids is not considered a risk for rabies transmission. The rabies virus cannot survive on surfaces in the environment for any substantial period of time. Such specific examples in healthcare settings include the following:
    - Touching a patient (unless an open wound, non-intact skin, or mucous membrane was contaminated with saliva or central nervous system material)
    - Changing a patient's bed linens
    - Taking a patient's blood pressure
    - Serving or cleaning up a patient's meals, including handling of used dishes and utensils
    - Phlebotomy (unless a needle stick injury occurs)
    - Handling the specimens of blood, cerebrospinal fluid (CSF), and urine of the patient in the laboratory
    - Presence near the operating or autopsy table during routine procedures
    - Observing or assisting with routine procedures

52. **Can a person donate blood when he is undergoing or has completed antirabies immunisation?**
Yes, he can donate blood but the blood recipient will not get protection against rabies through blood transfusion because the concentration of protective antibodies will be diluted.

53. **What is the clinical course of rabies in animals?**
The clinical course of rabies has three phases, namely, prodromal, excitatory, and paralytic stages. However, there is lot of variability of signs and lengths of these phases in animals.

54. **How do I suspect rabies in an animal?**
There are two forms of rabies illness seen in animals. One is known as the furious form and the other dumb form. In furious form, the animal can exhibit symptoms such as agitation and increased aggressiveness which is later followed by depression, paralysis, and death. The animals exhibiting the dumb form of rabies are lethargic, depressed, and eventually die. A change in animal's behaviour gives rise to suspicion of rabies. For example, a pet animal behaving as wild or a wild animal behaving tame should be suspected for rabies.

55. **What are the signs during the prodromal phase of rabies in animals?**
Prodromal phase may last for 1–3 days. The animal may show only vague nervous signs, which intensify rapidly. The disease progresses rapidly and death occurs within 10 days after the initial onset of signs. However, some animals may even die very rapidly without exhibiting marked clinical signs.

56. **What is furious form of rabies in animals?**
The excitatory phase following the prodromal phase is referred to as furious form of rabies. The animal becomes aggressive and may attack or bite. As the disease progresses, there is muscular incoordination, paralysis, and death.

57. **What is dumb form of rabies in animals?**
In dumb form of rabies, behavioural changes are minimal or absent. The animal is very quiet (not excited or aggressive) and may not generally attack or bite. The disease is manifested mainly by paralysis. Initially, there is paralysis of the throat and masseter muscles often causing profuse salivation and inability to swallow. Paralysis progresses rapidly and leads to death.

58. **Does a rabid dog show signs of hydrophobia (fear of water)?**
No, hydrophobia occurs in human beings not in dogs.

59. **Can rabies be transmitted to a dog due to eating the flesh of a dead rabid animal?**
Yes. In a rabid animal, rabies virus may be present in different organs. The dog can pick up the infection through oral mucous membrane.

60. **What are the symptoms of rabies in human beings?**
Rabies in human beings has two types of manifestations. The major one is the aggressive form in which there is hydrophobia (fear of water). The disease starts with headache, restlessness, fever, and itching at the site of bite. Subsequently, the patient develops fear of water, fear of air/breeze (aerophobia), fear of light (photophobia), excessive salivation, tremors, spasms, and convulsions. In the terminal stages, there is respiratory paralysis, cardiac arrest, and death in 1–5 days. The second, less common, form of the disease is the paralytic form. In this, there is gradual ascending paralysis, constipation, urinary retention, stupor, coma, and death. Hydrophobia is usually absent in these cases.

61. **How long does it take to show signs of rabies after being exposed?**
For rabies, the incubation period is more variable than with other infections. The incubation period in humans is usually several weeks to months, but ranges from days to years.

62. **How is rabies diagnosed?**
Laboratory tests can detect rabies virus in the saliva, skin, or brain tissue of a patient, but unfortunately, this is not possible until the disease has already progressed and it is too late for treatment. Therefore, the physician will most likely make a diagnosis based on the details of contact with a potentially infected animal and the likelihood of rabies infection from that. If the animal that has bitten is available for observation and testing, the diagnosis becomes easier.

63. **What do I need to do if a rabies outbreak has occurred?**
Contact public health officials. Avoid contact with animals that could have been exposed to rabies. Educate your family members about rabies and to avoid suspected animals.

64. **What steps should be taken if a person develops rabies?**
Immediate medical guidance should be sought.

65. **What steps should be taken for bite wound management?**
Wash the wound gently, preferably under running tap water, for at least 15 min. Apply detergent soap also. Apply povidone iodine, Dettol, Savlon, alcohol, etc. on the wound. Do not apply any irritant material like chilli powder, plant juices, herbal extracts, and pickles. Do not dress or bandage the wound. Seek medical guidance. A doctor will administer postexposure rabies vaccination/RIG, tetanus toxoid or anti-tetanus serum, antibiotics, etc. according to the severity of wound. Suturing of wound is generally avoided.

66. **Should animal bite wounds be washed?**
Washing bite wounds thoroughly with ample amount of clean running water and soap is very useful in washing away and inactivating the virus. Application of antiseptics, alcohol, etc. helps in inactivating the virus, thus reducing the chances of infection.

67. **Should the animal bite wounds be cauterised?**
No, cauterisation with carbolic acid or caustic agents should not be done. Rabies can be effectively prevented with modern antirabies vaccines.

68. **How does washing of wound help in protecting against rabies?**
Washing of wound under running tap water helps in washing away the virus from the site. It reduces the chances of infection.

69. **Will the washing of wound not cause abscess?**
Clean water is used for washing. Moreover, antiseptics are applied at the wound site and antibiotics are administered to prevent bacterial infection in the wound. Hence, washing should not be avoided.

70. **Why are the bite wounds not sutured?**
    Suturing is generally avoided because it may infect deeper tissues at the wound site with virus.
71. **What should be done if the wound is very extensive and it becomes necessary to suture the wound?**
    In case of an extensive wound, where suturing is essentially required, it should be done not immediately but after few hours. The suture should be loose and should not interfere with free bleeding and drainage. Infiltration of RIG at the wound site should be done before suturing is done.
72. **A pet dog of my neighbour bites me. What should I do?**
    Wash the wound immediately with soap or detergent in running tap water and apply any antiseptic. Go to a physician for further treatment. The doctor will assess the extent and severity of bite and accordingly will start the vaccination course and application of RIG (in Category III exposure). Keep the dog under observation for a period of 10 days or more for any kind of illness, abnormal behaviour, and death. Meanwhile continue taking vaccination dose on day 3 and day 7. If the dog remains healthy and alive till day 10 or afterwards, further vaccination may not be required, i.e. the 4th injection of vaccine due on day 14 is not required. If the dog dies, full course of vaccination should be taken.
73. **A stray dog bites me and runs away. What should I do?**
    Wash the wound immediately in running tap water with soap or detergent, apply any antiseptic, and go to the physician. After assessing the extent and severity of bite, the physician will administer RIG at wound site (in Category III exposure) and start vaccination course. Since the dog is not available for observation, full course of 5 injections of vaccine should be taken as per advice of the physician.
74. **Is not washing of bite wound at home ourselves harmful?**
    No, on the contrary, it helps in removal of virus from the site of bite and reduces chances of infection.
75. **How soon after an exposure should I seek medical attention?**
    Medical assistance should be obtained as soon as possible after an exposure to get timely PEP.
76. **What medical care do I need if I am exposed to rabies?**
    Thorough washing of the wound with soap and running water is the immediate effective method to decrease the chances of infection. Specific medical attention involves PEP that includes administration of antirabies vaccine and wherever necessary RIG as soon as possible after exposure.
77. **After I have been exposed, how long can I wait before getting postexposure vaccination?**
    You should seek postexposure vaccination as soon as possible. Do not wait.
78. **What does PEP consist of?**
    PEP consists of 5 doses of rabies vaccine given on treatment days 0, 3, 7, 14, and 28 in conjunction with a dose of RIG (depending on category of exposure). The vaccine is given intramuscularly, usually in the upper arm while RIG is infiltrated in and around the bite wound. If a person has previously received such vaccination or has taken pre-exposure vaccination against rabies, only 2 doses of vaccine (on days 0 and 3) will be given, and RIG is not required in such case.
79. **I have been told I need rabies vaccination. Do I need to start it immediately or should I wait for few days?**
    Rabies treatment should be started as soon as possible. The vaccine is highly effective if started well in time. However, if the vaccination could not be started promptly after the bite, the person should still receive the PEP treatment, no matter how much time has elapsed since the exposure.
80. **When a vaccinated pet dog bites a person, is it necessary to vaccinate the person?**
    It is advisable to vaccinate the person because it is difficult to ascertain the immune status of the dog at the time of biting. Secondly, in many cases, the pet dogs are not always kept restrained and under

supervision. So vaccination of the person is recommended to rule out any possibility of infection. However, vaccination can be discontinued if the dog remains healthy and alive after 10 days.

81. **What is the use of vaccinating a pet dog, if a person bitten by it still requires vaccination?**
Vaccination of pet dogs is done to protect it against contracting rabies from stray dogs and wild animals. Rabies is enzootic (widely prevalent) in stray animals and dog population in our country. Many times, it is also difficult to ascertain the date of the last rabies vaccination of a pet dog due to lack of any written record. Generally, facilities are not available to measure the level of protective antibodies in vaccinated dog at the time of bite. As rabies is a fatal disease, which cannot be reversed after onset, it is advisable to take no chance and start vaccination. However, vaccination can be discontinued if the dog remains healthy and alive after 10 days.

82. **Should I receive postexposure vaccination even for a small scratch or wound?**
Yes, if the animal was a suspect or confirmed rabid animal. You should consult your doctor to assess the risk.

83. **Can I just observe the dog for 10 days and not get vaccinated?**
No, it will subject you to serious risk. Dogs can shed rabies virus before showing clinical signs of rabies. In the event of a dog bite, washing of the wound with soap and water for at least 15 min should be immediately done and the advice of a medical expert should be sought. Vaccination should be initiated, and if the suspect dog is alive after 10 days, further doses of vaccination can be stopped.

84. **I was bitten by a dog 3 months ago and the dog died 4 days after it bit me. I have not taken any treatment. Am I at risk? What should I do?**
In areas where canine rabies is present, it is advisable to get PEP vaccination. The immunisation will protect you from the risk of developing rabies.

85. **People say that application of red chilli powder to the wound protects from rabies by destroying the virus. Is it correct?**
It is a misconception. Chilli powder, on the contrary, may be harmful. It causes irritation at the bite wound site and pushes the virus deeper into the tissue.

86. **Can a person bitten by a pet dog of his neighbours say that he does not need vaccination because he can observe the dog for 10 days?**
It is very risky. The person will be at risk of developing disease during this period. Once the disease progresses, it cannot be reversed. Therefore, vaccination should be started immediately, which can be stopped if the dog remains healthy and alive after 10 days.

87. **If a person does not take vaccination immediately after a stray dog bite, is it useful to start vaccination after a delay of 1 week or more?**
By not taking the vaccination and RIG, the person has put himself to risk all these days. But it is wise to get the treatment even at a late stage to stop the risk further. The treatment in such case is given as in a fresh case.

88. **Is it necessary to be vaccinated if the dog that bit me is alive?**
Dogs can shed rabies virus up to 10 days prior to showing clinical signs of disease. In areas where canine rabies is present, PEP vaccination should be initiated immediately. If the dog is alive up to 10 days after biting, the vaccination can be discontinued.

89. **Is there a possibility of survival of a person suffering from rabies?**
Death is almost certain in a patient of rabies (hydrophobia) after appearance of signs of the disease. Very few cases have been recorded where the persons recovered from the disease.

90. **Do herbal extracts, witchcraft, religious practices, and dietary restrictions cure rabies?**
No, these are only myths. Medical treatment should be given immediately to a person bitten by a rabid or suspected animal. Proper treatment only helps in prevention of rabies.

91. **How many injections of antirabies vaccine are required?**
The complete course of vaccination requires five injections. However, if the dog that has bitten a person is identified and remains healthy, normal, and alive 10 days after biting, the vaccination of the person can be discontinued.
92. **What is the schedule of antirabies vaccine injections?**
According to the WHO-approved schedule in India, the first dose is required immediately on the day of bite or at the first opportunity to get it (day 0). Subsequent four doses are given at day 3, day 7, day 14, and day 28. The sixth dose (optional, to be decided by the doctor) may be given on day 90.
93. **Is there any vaccine that can prevent rabies with only a single dose of vaccine?**
No, it is a misconception spread by untrained persons and quacks. Full course of vaccination under medical guidance can only prevent rabies.
94. **What is the site of injection of antirabies vaccine?**
Antirabies vaccine is given as intramuscular injection. It must be given into the muscles of the upper arm (deltoid region) in adults. In children with thin muscles in the arm, the injection is given into the anterolateral area of the thigh muscle. The vaccine should never be administered in the hip region.
95. **Why should antirabies vaccine injection be not given in the hip region?**
The vaccination is not done in the hip region (gluteal muscle) because high fat content in this area slows down the absorption of the vaccine.
96. **The doctor administered rabies vaccine into my buttocks, what do I do now?**
The vaccine should be re-administered correctly, in the deltoid area (arm).
97. **After a dog bite, a person received three doses of modern antirabies vaccine on day 0, day 3, and day 7. The dog was healthy till that time but it dies on day 8 or later. What should be done?**
The remaining two doses of vaccine should be taken at day 14 and day 28. The physician may also decide about the sixth optional dose at day 90 according to the case history.
98. **A person who had taken five injections of rabies vaccine after a dog bite is now bitten again. What should be done?**
Such person may need only two doses of modern rabies vaccine on day 0 and day 3. The application of RIG may not be required. Previously developed immunity of the person helps in raising the level of immunity further quickly. However, if the dog is suspected or confirmed for rabies, the physician may decide to give full course of vaccination to avoid any chance of disease.
99. **What should be done if I cannot take my next dose of rabies vaccine on a scheduled day?**
Consult your doctor. Rabies prevention is utmost important and changes should not be made in the schedule of doses.
100. **What do I do if I have missed a dose of vaccine on the prescribed date?**
The regimen should be followed as closely as possible. However, a 1- or 2-day deviation from the regimen may be acceptable. In case of longer delays, you should contact a physician so that he can evaluate the situation.
101. **I have received three doses of postexposure vaccination and the dog that bit me is still alive, should I continue with the vaccination and complete the entire course?**
There is no need to continue if the dog is still alive 10 days after biting.
102. **My baby was bitten by a suspect rabid animal, is he too young to get postexposure vaccination?**
No. Rabies vaccine is a life-saving vaccine and should not be withheld to anyone who has been exposed.
103. **I have been vaccinated previously with cell culture vaccine, and now I have been exposed to a rabid animal. Do I need to go through the full PEP vaccination regimen again?**
You will need only two booster doses of vaccine, given on day 0 and day 3. RIG administration is not needed in this case.

104. **I am immunocompromised, is it safe for me to get PEP vaccination?**
Yes. Rabies vaccine is a life-saving vaccine and should be given to anyone who has been exposed. If you are immunocompromised, you should receive PEP vaccination under the personal care of a physician.

105. **Can rabies vaccine be given to a patient with jaundice?**
Yes, it should be given. RIG if required (Category III) should be infiltrated. Antibody titre estimation is also recommended.

106. **What should be done if a person is taking antimalarial drugs, steroids, or immunosuppressive drugs?**
On day 0, two doses of vaccine should preferably be given at two different sites (upper arms, or thighs in young children). It is also desirable to administer RIG even in Category II exposures in such cases. The estimation of serum antibody titres should also be done on day 14 or later to ensure protection.

107. **Under what situations are two doses of rabies vaccine (instead of one) given on day 0?**
The first dose of the vaccine is doubled in the following situations:
   - The person comes for treatment after a delay of 48 h or more.
   - There are very extensive wounds in more risky parts of the body like head, neck, face, hands, and genitals due to bite by a suspect or confirmed rabid animal or by a wild animal like mongoose, jackal, and fox.
   - Patient is immunodeficient or suffering from AIDS.
   - Patient is taking immunosuppressive drugs, including corticosteroids, antimalarials, and anticancer drugs.
   - Patient is malnourished.
   - Patient is suffering from underlying chronic disease such as liver cirrhosis.
   - Patient has Category III exposure where administration of RIG is required but it is not available.

108. **I have a fever, should I wait to receive postexposure vaccination?**
No. Rabies vaccine is a life-saving vaccine. You should receive postexposure vaccination under the personal care of a physician.

109. **People acquire immunity against other viral infections, but why is it not so when rabies infection occurs due to bite?**
When an infected animal bites a person, the virus from the site of bite enters a nerve and then travels to the central nervous system (spinal cord, brain) through the nerves. Thus, the virus does not come in blood, i.e. there is no viraemia which is required for the normal immune mechanism of the body to function. The antibody production starts only when the virus from the brain goes to different organs through nerves. But it happens too late at a stage when the patient's brain has already been severely affected. The patient dies soon due to respiratory paralysis or due to cardiac arrest.

110. **Are antirabies vaccines and RIG one and the same thing?**
No, they are quite different. Antirabies vaccine gives protection by producing antibodies in the body against rabies virus. It produces active immunity and takes some time to do so. RIG on the other hand is a ready-made antibody against rabies virus which inactivates the virus immediately at the site. It provides passive immunity to prevent infection.

111. **In case of a dog bite, should one prefer antirabies vaccine or RIG?**
There is no question of preference. Both have different purposes. Depending upon the site and extent of bite wound, the doctor decides whether antirabies vaccine alone is required or is it to be given along with local infiltration of RIG. In case of severe bite exposures (Category III exposures), antirabies vaccination as well as local application of RIG is required for complete protection.

112. **What is the added advantage of giving RIG in addition to vaccine?**

RIG is a ready-made antibody against rabies virus and can provide immediate passive immunity. Its local infiltration in bite wounds helps in neutralising the virus present in wound and thus prevents entry of the virus into a nerve ending at the site of bite. In contrast to this, the development of active immunity from vaccine takes some time, and the desired protective level of antibody may occur by day 14 after initiating the vaccination with modern vaccines. However, in severe bite cases or when the bite is close to brain, the disease may develop before the protective immunity develops. RIG thus provides passive protection during this initial period when the active immunity is still developing.

113. **Is it essential to take the course of rabies vaccine even when RIG has been administered immediately after bite?**
Yes, RIG is not a substitute to vaccine. RIG and vaccine both have different specific purposes. The purpose of RIG is to provide immediate short-term passive protection while the vaccine is given to develop immunity for protection against the disease during later periods.

114. **If a patient of Category III exposure is given only rabies vaccination but RIG is not administered locally, should immunoglobulin be infiltrated afterwards?**
RIG should be infiltrated locally into the wounded tissues before beginning the vaccination. However, many times it is not done due to unavailability of immunoglobulin or ignorance. Administering immunoglobulin after the development of antibody response due to vaccination may affect the immunity produced by the vaccination. The physician has to evaluate the situation, taking into consideration the time gap after the vaccination and decide accordingly.

115. **RIG is not available where I live, is there an alternative?**
There is no alternative to RIG. In developing countries, it is generally available in larger cities. If there is a delay in finding RIG, you should begin the vaccination series immediately and seek RIG elsewhere if possible. You can receive RIG up to 7 days after initiating the postexposure vaccination.

116. **What should be done if RIG is unavailable or the patient is unable to afford it?**
In such cases, the wound management acquires much greater importance. The wound must be thoroughly flushed with povidone iodine or surgical spirit to inactivate the virus. Further, the patient should preferably be given two doses of vaccine on day 0 in both deltoids.

117. **What should be the time gap between RIG and vaccination?**
Both should be given on the day 0, i.e. immediately after the bite. RIG may be infiltrated in and around the bite wound first. The vaccine should be injected within about 1 h after administering RIG.

118. **Can RIG be given after starting vaccination?**
Ideally the RIG should be administered at the earliest after the bite, preferably on day 0 and at the same time when the first dose of vaccine is injected. However, in case of its unavailability or certain other circumstances, it may be administered within 72 h of starting of vaccine. Administration of RIG much beyond the start of vaccination may hamper the development of immunity by the vaccine. The physician has to take appropriate decision after evaluating the actual situation.

119. **What is the site of injecting RIG?**
RIG is infiltrated directly into and around the wounds. The leftover RIG, if any, after adequate wound infiltration can be given IM into the anterolateral thigh at a site away from the site of rabies vaccine injection. It should not be injected into the gluteal region.

120. **Is there any special technique to administer RIG locally in the wound?**
Yes, certain precautions are to be taken and it requires some experience as well. The RIG should be brought to room temperature (after removing it from refrigerator) before injecting. It should be administered with sterile hypodermic syringe with 26 G nee-

dle carefully into and around all wounds to locally neutralise the virus. Care should be taken to cause minimal traumatisation. If the wounds are extensive, the RIG can be diluted to increase its volume to cover whole of the wounded area. Any leftover RIG should be given by deep IM injection at a site away from the vaccine site.

121. **What is the dose of RIG?**
The dose rates of human rabies immunoglobulin (HRIG) and equine rabies immunoglobulin (ERIG) are different. HRIG is given at the rate of 20 IU/kg bodyweight. Its maximum dose is 1,500 IU or 10 ml. The dosage of ERIG is 40 IU/kg bodyweight with a maximum of 3,000 IU or 10 ml.

122. **What is the difference between ERIG and HRIG?**
ERIG is equine RIG and is produced in horses. HRIG is human RIG and is produced in humans. Both contain antibodies against rabies virus but the dose of ERIG is 40 IU/Kg bodyweight while that of HRIG it is 20 IU/Kg bodyweight.

123. **How do we calculate the total dose of RIG administration?**
The dose of ERIG is 40 IU/Kg bodyweight and the total maximum dose is 3,000 IU or 10 ml. HRIG is administered at the rate of 20 IU/Kg bodyweight and the total maximum dose is 1,500 IU or 10 ml. The concentration (IU/ml) and the volume of RIG in a vial may differ in different brands of RIG. In case of a vial of ERIG containing 300 IU per ml, the total dose of ERIG in ml will be equal to $1/300 \times 40$ IU $\times$ bodyweight in Kg. Similarly, the total dose in ml in case of a vial of HRIG containing 150 IU per ml will be calculated as $1/150 \times 20$ IU $\times$ bodyweight in Kg.

124. **Is ERIG safe?**
Generally, the currently available ERIG is purified and safe but rarely there may be adverse reactions ranging from serum sickness like reaction to anaphylaxis. Hence, it is always safer to be ready for emergency situations and to keep emergency kits on hand. ERIG should preferably be given in a hospital equipped with adequate facilities.

125. **What are the signs of adverse reaction after administration of antirabies serum or ERIG?**
The immediate adverse reactions are anaphylactic type. The signs include hypotension, dyspnoea, syncope, and urticaria. Serious type of anaphylactic shock is rare. Serum sickness consisting of inflammatory reactions (type III hypersensitivity reaction) may occur after 6 days in some cases. It causes fever, pruritus, rash, urticaria, adenopathy, and arthralgia.

126. **Can adverse reactions occur with ERIG even after a negative skin test?**
In some patients, even after a negative skin test, there may be adverse reactions with ERIG. These reactions may range from serum sickness like reaction to anaphylaxis. Hence, it is always safer to be ready for emergency situations and to keep emergency kits on hand. ERIG should preferably be given in an appropriately equipped hospital.

127. **Is the adverse reaction due to ERIG or antirabies serum curable?**
Yes, the adverse reactions/emergencies can be managed in a well-equipped medical centre. Anaphylactic shock can be managed with adrenaline, oxygen, artificial respiration, hydrocortisone, and antihistamines. Serum sickness can be treated with nonsteroidal anti-inflammatory agents and antihistamines.

128. **If a patient shows positive skin test to ERIG, what should be done?**
In such cases, administration of ERIG may not be safe, so it is advisable to administer HRIG, which is practically safe. However, if the patient cannot afford HRIG and the situation is life threatening, ERIG may be given under strict medical supervision and after adopting appropriate measures/medication to prevent any emergency in a fully equipped medical facility. It is also advisable to inform the patient about the risk involved and to obtain his written consent.

129. **What should be done if the wounds are extensive but the volume of RIG is inadequate to infiltrate the wounds thoroughly?**
RIG can be diluted with normal saline to increase its volume to infiltrate all wounds. Any leftover RIG should be injected in the thigh (away from the vaccine site) by IM route.

130. **What is the difference between pre-exposure and postexposure prophylaxis?**
Pre-exposure vaccination is given prior to an exposure in which antirabies vaccine is administered to the people who are at higher risk of exposure to rabies. Postexposure vaccination is given after an exposure to rabies has occurred. It involves administration of rabies vaccine along with or without RIG according to the exposure-risk category.

131. **Should I get a preventive rabies vaccine before being exposed?**
People who are at higher risk of being exposed to rabies may get the vaccine before exposure to rabies. The general public normally does not require pre-exposure rabies vaccination.

132. **Who should get pre-exposure vaccination against rabies?**
   - Rabies vaccine is recommended for the following groups of persons:
   - Persons of who are at greater risk of exposure, such as veterinarians, animal handlers, stray dog control personnel, and certain laboratory workers
   - Persons whose activities bring them in frequent contact with rabies virus or potentially rabid bats, raccoons, skunks, cats, dogs, or other species at risk for having rabies
   - International travellers who are likely to come in contact with animals in areas where dog rabies is common, especially if there is likelihood of limited access to appropriate medical care

133. **What is the use of pre-exposure vaccination in pet owners?**
Due to the endemic nature of rabies in India and close contact with pet animals, the animal lovers and pet owners constitute a high-risk group. Pre-exposure vaccination protects them against rabies, and in case of an exposure, such persons may not need RIG and require less number of postexposure vaccine injections.

134. **After getting pre-exposure vaccination, am I protected if I am bitten by a dog?**
No, pre-exposure vaccination does not eliminate the need for additional therapy after a rabies exposure. It, however, simplifies the postexposure treatment by eliminating the need of RIG administration and decreasing the number of rabies vaccine doses.

135. **I am engaged in the work of animal handling and control. I have been recommended pre-exposure vaccination against rabies. How does pre-exposure vaccination differ from the postexposure vaccination?**
Pre-exposure vaccination is given before any exposure in order to develop immunity against rabies in advance before any exposure occurs. Postexposure vaccination is given after the exposure (e.g. dog bite) occurs. Pre-exposure vaccination helps in reducing the risk from an unapparent exposure and also reduces the number of doses of postexposure vaccination after an exposure takes place.

136. **Is an immunised person totally protected if bitten by a rabid animal?**
No, he may be only partially protected. A vaccinated person should receive two more doses of postexposure rabies vaccine: one dose immediately (day 0) and one three days later (day 3).

137. **What is the advantage of being immunised against rabies in advance (pre-exposure vaccination) if I still have to receive additional doses of vaccine if I am bitten by an animal?**
Pre-exposure vaccination simplifies the postexposure treatment. It eliminates the need of RIG and decreases the number of vaccine injections after an exposure. This is important in high-risk group of people. Pre-exposure vaccination might also provide

protection against unknown exposures to rabies.

138. **How often do I need to get a booster after pre-exposure vaccination?**
Periodic booster injections are recommended for persons who are at continuous or frequent risk of exposure. If their rabies virus-neutralising antibody titres fall below 0.5 IU/ml, they should receive one routine booster. For people who are potentially at risk of laboratory exposure to high concentrations of live rabies virus, antibody testing should be done every 6 months while those not at continual risk of exposure should have serological monitoring every 2 years.

139. **I am planning to keep a pet dog at my home. Should all of my family members receive pre-exposure vaccination?**
No. You should ensure that your dog is vaccinated with an effective canine rabies vaccine before bringing it home. It should also be regularly vaccinated subsequently as per schedule. You should teach your family, especially children, how to treat the dog properly and to tell a parent if they are bitten.

140. **What kinds of antirabies vaccines are available?**
Several types of vaccines produced by different agencies are available. These include human diploid cell culture vaccine (HDCV), purified chick embryo cell vaccine (PCEC), purified duck embryo vaccine (PDEV), and purified Vero cell rabies vaccine (PVRV).

141. **Several brands of modern vaccines are currently available in the market. What is the difference between them?**
These vaccines are produced by different agencies, but all approved vaccines are protective. These vaccines may differ in production technique, amount of dose in each injection, and stability at high temperature.

142. **There are several types of modern antirabies vaccines in the market. Which one is preferable?**
All modern vaccines approved by the government are safe and effective. However, the doctor may prefer a particular type (brand) of vaccine based on the situation and his experience.

143. **What is the difference between cell culture vaccine (CCV) and nervous tissue vaccine (NTV)?**
CCV is produced in cell lines and is highly purified and among the most efficacious vaccines. NTV is usually crude vaccine made by infecting sheep or goats with rabies virus and harvesting their brain tissue to produce vaccine. The course of vaccination with CCV is short but the course of NTV is long, painful, and not always as effective. Side effects are more often reported in persons who receive NTV than in those that receive CCV. The side effects from NTV can be very serious including paralysis, whereas side effects of CTV are extremely rare and only very minor. WHO strongly advocates the use of CCV and recommends complete discontinuation of the production and use of NTV.

144. **If a person is allergic to egg, can he be safely injected with purified chick embryo or duck embryo vaccine?**
Though these vaccines have high degree of purity, there is a theoretical and remote risk of allergic reaction in a person who is allergic to avian proteins. In such persons, other vaccines like human diploid cell culture vaccine or purified Vero cell rabies vaccine should be used to avoid any such reaction.

145. **What does potency of vaccine mean?**
The potency is the capacity of the vaccine to induce immune response. WHO recommends that rabies vaccine potency should be 2.5 IU or more/dose.

146. **Some people say that antirabies vaccination is painful and dangerous. Is it so?**
This is a myth in context with the modern rabies vaccines. The modern rabies vaccines are safe and painless. There is nothing to fear about these. However, in earlier days, the old neural tissue vaccines were prepared from animal brain tissue which could sometimes cause side effects. Moreover, the old vaccines required more number of injections and the procedure was not quite painless.

That is why the people may get carried away by the old notions.

147. **β-propiolactone used for inactivation of vaccine is a known carcinogen. Is it safe to inject vaccine containing β-propiolactone?**
Yes, it is quite safe. β-propiolactone loses its carcinogenicity during the process of inactivation of rabies virus. Its final concentration is very less. Hence, it is safe and there is no reason to worry.

148. **Is there any antirabies vaccine that gives lifelong protection?**
There is no such vaccine which gives lifelong immunity. Every time a person is exposed to an animal bite, he needs to consult a physician for proper protective immunisation.

149. **Are there any adverse reactions of rabies vaccine?**
Adverse reactions to modern rabies vaccine and RIG are not common. Mild local reactions to the rabies vaccine, such as pain, redness, swelling, or itching at the injection site, have been reported. Rarely, symptoms such as headache, nausea, abdominal pain, muscle aches, and dizziness have been reported. Local pain and low-grade fever may follow injection of RIG.

150. **Under what circumstances rabies vaccination should not be done?**
Vaccination is essential for prevention of rabies. Once the disease develops, it cannot be reversed and it is always fatal. Hence, it should not be avoided under any circumstances.

151. **What precautions are needed while buying vaccine and carrying it?**
Buy the vaccine from a reliable medical store which has continuously good facility of storing vaccines in refrigerators. Hold the vaccine at low temperature while transporting too. Use icebox or a thermos flask with ice for carrying vaccine.

152. **How should the vaccine be stored at home?**
The vaccine should be kept in a refrigerator at 2–8 °C, not in the freezing (ice-forming) chamber.

153. **What happens if by mistake the rabies vaccine is kept in the freezing chamber of a refrigerator?**
Freezing and subsequent thawing of the vaccine affects the potency of the vaccine. Do not use such vaccine.

154. **Can the vaccine cause rabies?**
No.

155. **Can a person change over from one type of cell culture vaccine to another during the vaccination schedule?**
It should be preferred to have all doses of same type of vaccine.

156. **What can be the reasons for shifting from one type of vaccine to another after the first vaccination dose?**
Price difference, sudden unavailability of one brand, and manifestation of allergy to a particular type of vaccine are some reasons leading to the change of type of vaccine during the course of vaccination.

157. **Can a pregnant woman receive rabies vaccine if exposed to rabies?**
Yes, she definitely needs to be protected against rabies disease. No foetal abnormalities have been reported with the rabies vaccine. She can even receive routine pre-exposure vaccination against rabies if her risk of exposure is high.

158. **Can a mother with a breastfed baby be given antirabies vaccine?**
Yes, antirabies vaccines are inactivated vaccines. These can be given to the lactating mothers and have no bad effect on the breastfed baby.

159. **Can antirabies vaccine be given to a child suffering from chicken pox or measles?**
Yes, it can be given and it is protective. It should not be avoided on the pretext of fever, because it will endanger the child with risk of rabies.

160. **Can antirabies vaccine be given to HIV or AIDS patients?**
Yes, but such patients have less body immunity status. Therefore, on day 0, they may require two injections of vaccine instead of one. Two doses of vaccine are injected at two different sites (upper arms, or thighs in

young children). It is also desirable to administer RIG even in Category II exposures. The estimation of serum antibody titres should also be done on day 14 or later to ensure protection.

161. **Is the dose of antirabies vaccine different in the newborn babies, infants, young children, and adults?**
The dose of antirabies vaccine is same for all age groups. It does not differ with body size.

162. **Can antirabies vaccine be given along with other vaccines?**
Yes, it can be given with other vaccines. However, it should not be mixed with other vaccines and should be given at the recommended site (upper arm, or thigh in young children) and at a site different from other vaccine.

163. **Do some drugs interfere with the production of immunity with rabies vaccine?**
Antimalarial drugs, steroids, and immunosuppressive drugs may affect the efficacy of rabies vaccines.

164. **Is there any dietary restriction during PEP course of vaccination?**
It is generally advisable to avoid consuming alcohol during the antirabies vaccine administration as it may affect the immune response.

165. **Can I drink alcohol during the course of antirabies vaccination?**
Excessive consumption of alcohol should be avoided.

166. **I was bitten by a dog. Now, I am receiving rabies vaccination. Can I transmit rabies to other people?**
A person cannot transmit rabies to other people unless he develops clinical signs of rabies. The vaccination you are receiving will protect you from developing rabies, and therefore, you pose no rabies-related risk to other people.

167. **What is the difference between intramuscular administration and intradermal administration of cell culture rabies vaccine?**
The route and dose of vaccine administration are different in these two methods of vaccination. The purpose is same. Intramuscular vaccination is usually done by all physicians but intradermal vaccination may require some particular skill and training.

168. **Can we change the route of vaccination from intramuscular to intradermal or vice versa during the course of vaccination?**
The route of vaccination, either intramuscular to intradermal, should ideally remain the same throughout the course of vaccination in a patient.

169. **Can we shift from one type of vaccine to another during the course of intradermal rabies vaccination?**
As far as possible, the same vaccine should be used throughout the course of vaccination.

170. **Is it essential to check the efficacy of intradermal vaccination by testing serum for rabies antibodies?**
The intradermal vaccination is well tested and WHO approved. Hence, it is not essential to carry out the test for rabies antibodies levels routinely.

171. **The intramuscular dose of some antirabies vaccines is 1 ml while that of some others is 0.5 ml, but the intradermal dosage of all vaccines is uniformly 0.1 ml. Is it so?**
Yes, the intradermal dose of all approved vaccines is uniformly 0.1 ml per intradermal site.

172. **Is it essential to follow the schedule of intradermal vaccination strictly?**
The first three doses of intradermal vaccination on days 0, 3, and 7 are very crucial and should be given as close to the scheduled days and preferably completed by day 7. However, for the fourth dose on day 28, 1–2 days of variation may be acceptable.

173. **Are there any contraindications to intradermal vaccination?**
The intradermal vaccination is contraindicated when the patient is immunocompromised or is on chloroquine or any

immunosuppressant therapy (anticancer drugs, radiation therapy, long-term steroid usage, etc.). In such cases, rabies vaccines should be given by intramuscular route.

174. **Are there any dietary restrictions during intradermal vaccination?**
There are no dietary restrictions during intradermal vaccination.

175. **Is intradermal vaccination contraindicated in pregnancy and lactation?**
No, it is not contraindicated in these situations.

176. **Are the modern antirabies vaccines always protective?**
The modern vaccines are very immunogenic and protective but the protection may fail under certain circumstances.

177. **What are the reasons for failure of antirabies vaccination?**
Some cases of rabies are reported despite antirabies vaccination. There may be several reasons for this. It may be due to insufficient wound treatment, non-administration of RIG by infiltration immediately at the site of bite in Category III exposures, incomplete infiltration of RIG in all wounds, use of poorly stored vaccine, delay in vaccination, faulty vaccination in hip muscles instead of arm, incomplete vaccination course, immunodeficiency of the person, use of some other drugs simultaneously, etc.

178. **What is the method of confirmation of protection after immunisation?**
It requires measuring the level of rabies virus-neutralising antibody in blood serum after administration of vaccine. Antibody titre of 0.5 IU/ml in serum is considered protective. Some select centres/laboratories have this facility.

179. **Is it essential to carry out antibody test on all the patients after vaccination?**
Antibody tests are not required routinely if the vaccine is maintained at low (refrigeration) temperature and the vaccination is done according to the approved schedule and correct method.

180. **How can I protect my pet from rabies?**
Get your pet dogs and cats vaccinated on regular basis. Keep your pets indoors and under your supervision. Spay or neuter your pets to limit the number of your pets so that they are manageable. Arrange stray animal control in your neighbourhood.

181. **Why does my pet need rabies vaccine?**
Your pets and other domestic animals can be infected when they are bitten by rabid stray or wild animals. Pets should therefore be vaccinated to prevent rabies infection in them and its further transmission to human beings.

182. **What is the pre-exposure vaccination schedule for pet dogs and cats?**
Pre-exposure immunisation of pet dogs and cats is recommended on a routine basis. First dose is given at the age of 3 months or above. If primary vaccination is given prior to 3 months age, a repeat vaccination (secondary) must be given at the age of 3 months. Thereafter, annual booster dose is recommended in areas where rabies is endemic.

183. **Postexposure vaccination is required in the bitten person even when the biting animal is a vaccinated pet dog. What is the use of regular vaccination of pet dogs then?**
Vaccination of the dog protects it against rabies from the stray or wild animals. However, since the protection status of the vaccinated dog is not confirmed by testing, it is recommended to vaccinate the exposed person to prevent any risk.

184. **What should be done if an unvaccinated or partially vaccinated pet dog is bitten by a stray dog?**
If the stray dog is suspected to be rabid, it is advisable to consult the veterinarian and arrange euthanasia (painless death) of the pet dog. But if the rabid status of the stray dog is not known, the bite wound should be immediately washed with a detergent soap and cold water followed by application of antiseptics. This should be followed by immediate postexposure vaccination of the pet. The pet dog should be confined to an isolated place and kept under careful observation for at least 2 months (or even up to 6

months) for development of possible signs of rabies.

185. **What should be done if a pet dog is bitten by a stray dog?**
Thoroughly wash the wound with a detergent soap. Apply some antiseptic and consult a veterinarian immediately.

186. **What should be done if a vaccinated dog is bitten by a rabid animal?**
PEP vaccination in such cases is not very successful; hence, ideally, such dog should be euthanised (humanely killed) by a veterinarian.

187. **What should be done if a vaccinated pet dog dies suddenly?**
It is advisable to consult the veterinarian and arrange post-mortem examination of the dog for ruling out or confirmation of rabies. If is not possible, it should be considered a suspect case and all those who had come in contact with the saliva of the animal (directly or through its fomites) should be given postexposure vaccination.

188. **What should be done to the animal that has bitten a person?**
It is important to know whether the animal at the time of biting was rabid or not. If the biting animal is a pet or can be safely caught, it should be confined at an isolated place and kept under observation for at least 10 days. If it remains healthy for 10 days after the bite, it is considered not rabid at the time of the bite; however, if it develops disease or dies within this period, it is suspected as rabid.

189. **What should be done if my pet dog or cat is bitten by a wild animal?**
Any animal bitten or scratched by a wild carnivorous mammal should be regarded as having been exposed to rabies. Unvaccinated dogs and cats exposed to a rabid animal should be euthanised immediately. If the owner is unwilling to have this done, the animal should be placed in strict isolation for 6 months and vaccinated 1 month before being released. Animals with expired vaccinations need to be evaluated on a case-by-case basis. Dogs and cats that are currently vaccinated are kept under observation for 45 days.

190. **I am moving to a rabies-free country and want to take my pets with me. What should I do?**
The details of regulation about importing pets into rabies-free countries vary by country. Check with the embassy of your destination country.

191. **Why should we be concerned about rabies in wildlife?**
Rabies is a serious public health concern because if left untreated it is always fatal. In the regions where rabies in pet or domestic animals has already been controlled, there is risk of transmission of infection from wildlife to domestic animals and human beings. Further, in suburban and rural areas, there are more chances of interaction with wildlife, increasing the risk of rabies exposure.

192. **What is oral rabies vaccine (ORV) bait?**
ORV baits are generally used in targeted areas to vaccinate the wildlife species, such as foxes, raccoons, and coyotes, by oral route to prevent the spread of rabies. ORV bait consists of a sachet or plastic packet containing rabies vaccine. To make the baits attractive to wildlife, the baits are either waxed to the inside of a fishmeal or dog meal outer shell or covered with fishmeal crumbs.

193. **How does a wild animal (raccoon, coyote, grey fox) get vaccinated by eating the ORV bait?**
The vaccine contained inside a plastic packet is enclosed in an edible bait material. When an animal eats the bait, the vaccine packet inside is punctured allowing the animal to swallow the vaccine. The animal's immune system is then activated and it makes antibodies to fight the disease.

194. **Is ORV bait available for vaccinating dogs in India?**
No.

195. **Can I use the ORV bait to vaccinate my dog or cat?**
No. This vaccine is generally approved for use in wildlife and may not be approved for pets in your area. Your pet should be

vaccinated by a veterinarian in accordance with the approved methods and local laws.

196. **What if my dog or cat eats an ORV bait?** This vaccine has been shown to be safe in more than 60 different species of animals, including domestic dogs and cats. Eating a large number of baits may cause a temporarily upset stomach in your pet, but it does not pose a long-term health risk. Do not attempt to remove the bait from your pet; doing so may cause you to be bitten and could lead to vaccine exposure. If your pet becomes ill from bait consumption, contact your veterinarian.

197. **How long does the immunity from vaccine last?** Research suggests this vaccine should be effective for more than a year; however, it is difficult to determine how immune systems in individual animals will respond to the vaccine.

198. **How long do ORV baits last in the environment?** Studies have shown that most baits are eaten within 4 days, and almost all baits are gone in 1 week. If baits are not found and eaten, they will dissolve exposing the vaccine packet. Sunlight and exposure to air inactivates the vaccine.

199. **What should I do if I find ORV bait in my house premises?** After wearing gloves, you may remove the bait and put it in some area having thick plantation. Wild animals are likely to visit that area and take up the bait. Alternatively, you may put it in a bag and dispose it of in the garbage disposal bin. Then wash your hands thoroughly with soap and water.

200. **How are ORV baits distributed in cities and suburban areas?** Oral baits in urban and suburban areas are generally distributed by hand by the specialised personnel. However, in some countries, baits are distributed in rural or open areas using aircraft.

About the Author

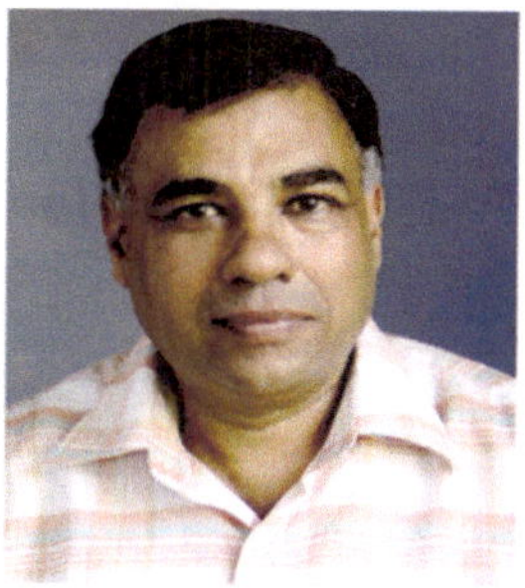

Dr. Sudhi Ranjan Garg is a senior Professor of Veterinary Public Health and Epidemiology in Lala Lajpat Rai University of Veterinary and Animal Sciences at Hisar (India). He has also worked as Head of the Department. Dr. Garg obtained the degree of Bachelor of Veterinary Sciences and Animal Husbandry in 1979. He was awarded a national level Junior Research Scholarship by the Indian Council of Agricultural Research and obtained the degree of Master of Veterinary Sciences in Veterinary Public Health and Epidemiology in 1982. He was later awarded Russian Government Scholarship for doctoral studies and obtained Ph.D. from the prestigious All Russian Institute of Experimental Veterinary Medicine in Moscow in 1991. Dr. Garg has over 30 years experience in graduate and postgraduate teaching and research. He works as a subject matter specialist for many organizations. Recognizing his expertise, the Indian Association of Veterinary Public Health Specialists has elected Dr. Garg as its Fellow.

Actively working with the Alliance for Rabies Control (UK), Global Alliance for Rabies Control (USA), and the Commonwealth Veterinary Association, Dr. Garg regularly coordinates educational rabies campaigns for raising community awareness, particularly among schoolchildren, college students, pet owners, farmers and urban people. The Global Alliance for Rabies Control commending his zealous work has cited him as an example of "Local Heroes" who have taken action towards rabies prevention and control efforts in their country. Dr. Garg also works as resource faculty in the Continuing Veterinary Education Programme run by the Veterinary Council of India to train the State Veterinary Officers on rabies diagnosis, prevention and control.

Dr. Garg is currently busy in pushing forward the 'One Health' concept in the region. He has

S.R. Garg, *Rabies in Man and Animals*, DOI 10.1007/978-81-322-1605-6, over 100 scientific papers and several books to his credit. His earlier books include *Understanding Rabies and its Prevention*, *Interdisciplinary Approach for Tuberculosis Control*, *Environmental Security: Human and Animal Health*, *Human and Animal Health: Environmental Perspectives*, *Veterinary and Livestock Sector: A Blueprint for Capacity Building*, and *Handbook of Quality Control of Dairy and Meat Products*.

Index

S.R. Garg, *Rabies in Man and Animals*, DOI 10.1007/978-81-322-1605-6,